AF396675

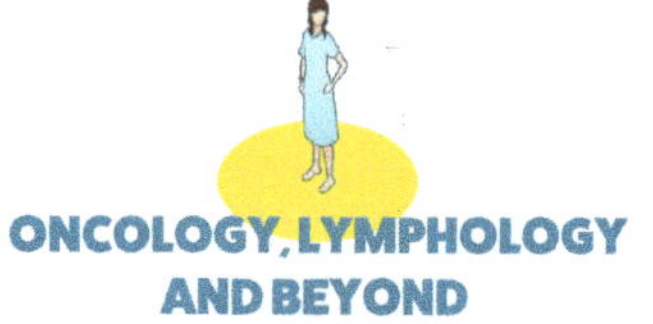

ONCOLOGY, LYMPHOLOGY
AND BEYOND

NICK GEBRUERS & HANNE VERBELEN

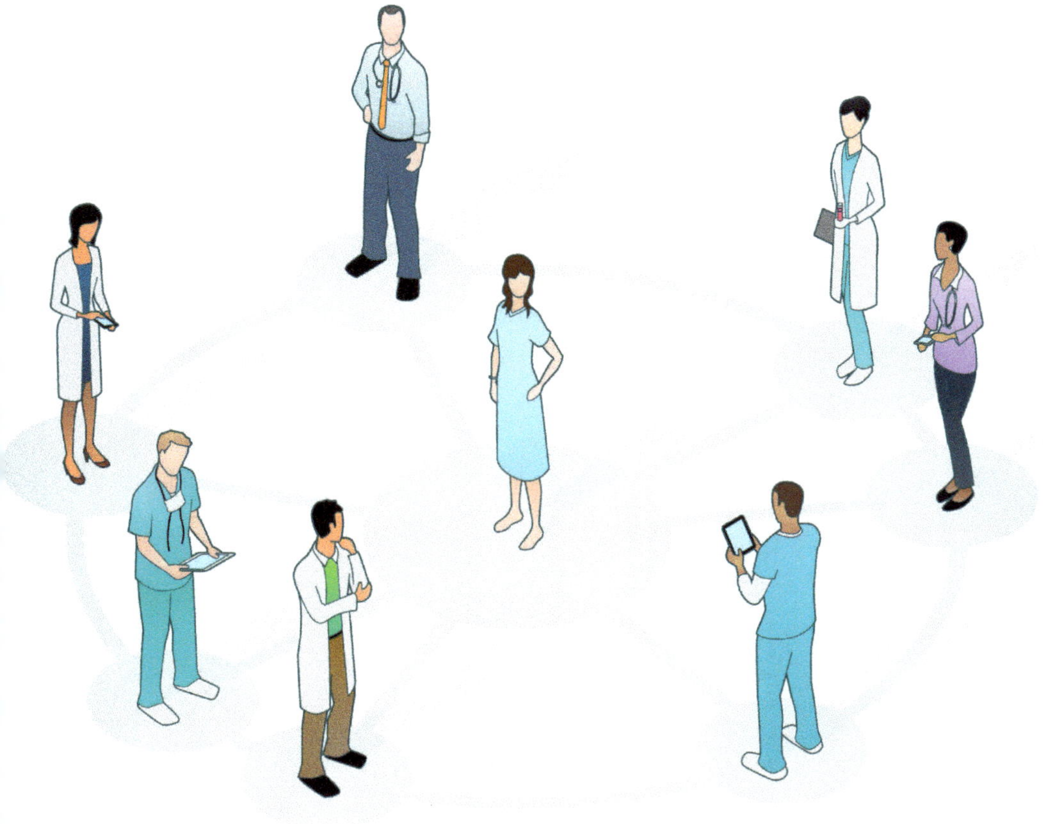

ONCOLOGY, LYMPHOLOGY AND BEYOND

PATIENT-CENTRED CARE FROM A PHYSIOTHERAPEUTIC POINT OF VIEW

acco learn

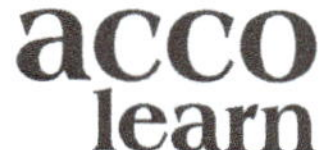

First edition: 2021

Published by
Acco cv, Sluisstraat 10, 3000 Leuven, Belgium
E-mail: uitgeverij@acco.be – Website: www.acco.be

The Netherlands:
Acco Uitgeverij, Westvlietweg 67 F, 2495 AA Den Haag, The Netherlands
E-mail: info@uitgeverijacco.nl – Website: www.accouitgeverij.nl

Cover design: Frisco-ontwerpbureau
Typesetting: Crius Group

D/2021/0543/249   NUR 860   ISBN 978-94-6414-435-2

DIGITAL STUDY MATERIAL

The edition Oncology, lymphology and beyond includes:

- this paper handbook
- digital study material

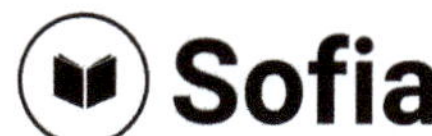

Access to the digital study material:

1. Surf to www.sofialearn.com/app. If you already have a Sofia account, log in. If you do not yet have a Sofia account, you can make one by clicking on the button 'sign up' and filling in your details. Once you have done this, click on 'complete registration'. You will then receive an e-mail at the e-mail address you have given. You can confirm the opening of your account by clicking on the button 'confirm registration' in the e-mail.
2. In the online learning platform, you must click on the button 'add course' in the blue navigation bar on the left-hand side. On the page that opens, you can enter the code below. This will give you access to the digital study material.

3. Are you a student? Choose your 'portal' or 'virtual class'. (No portal yet? Ask your teacher about it!)

Attention! Every code is unique, strictly personal and can only be changed just once. Every code therefore gives you lifelong access to the course and, consequently, does not need to be renewed.

What if you are not able to make an account or change the code?

You can ask for help from our help desk by filling in the contact form on our contact page (www.sofialearn.com/app/contact). The help desk will contact you as soon as possible.

Are you a teacher?

If you are a teacher, but not the author of this edition, and would like to know more about the possibilities as a teacher for using this online course, please get in touch with us by filling in the contact form (www.sofialearn.com/app/contact) or by e-mailing us on infosofia@acco.be.

CONTENT

AUTHORS

Dr. Nick Gebruers (1976), physical therapist, is Professor of Rehabilitation Sciences and Physiotherapy (REVAKI-MOVANT) at the University of Antwerp. His field of research is edema treatment. He has authored > 50 publications on the topic. His teaching activities are mainly situated in research sciences and vascular rehabilitation. He is cofounder of oedema.be and a scientific collaborator at the multidisciplinary edema clinic of the Antwerp University Hospital.

Dr. Hanne Verbelen (1988), physical therapist, is an educational expert in the Department of Rehabilitation Sciences and Physiotherapy (REVAKI-MOVANT) at the University of Antwerp. As a researcher she is active in the field of breast cancer related morbidity, including lymphedema and breast edema. Her teaching activities are mainly situated in the domain of oncological rehabilitation and lymphology, with a strong focus on blended learning.

Dr. Jill Meirte (1982), physical therapist, finished a PhD on scar assessments and physiotherapeutic treatments for scars in collaboration with *Oscare*, a (burn) scar after-care and research centre located in Antwerp. She combines research activities with coordinating and teaching responsibilities in the Department of Rehabilitation Sciences and Physiotherapy (REVAKI-MOVANT) at the University of Antwerp. Her teaching activities cover topics such as the International Classification of Functioning, Disability and Health (ICF) and burn and scar care. She is an ICF trainer and has special interest and clinical experience in non-invasive physical scar management, patient-reported outcome measures and digitalizing PT care (e-health). She strives towards a *'scarless'* world and patient-centred care.

Mrs. Timia Van Soom (PhD student) (1991), physical therapist, is a graduate teaching and research assistant at the Department of Rehabilitation Sciences and Physiotherapy of the University of Antwerp (REVAKI-MOVANT). Her doctoral research focuses on the impact of cancer treatments on energy metabolism and related comorbidities during and after treatment. Her teaching activities are mainly situated in the domain of human physiology and oncological rehabilitation. She is an active member of the Flemish Interuniversity Research group on Rehabilitation in Internal Diseases (FIRRI).

1 INTRODUCTION

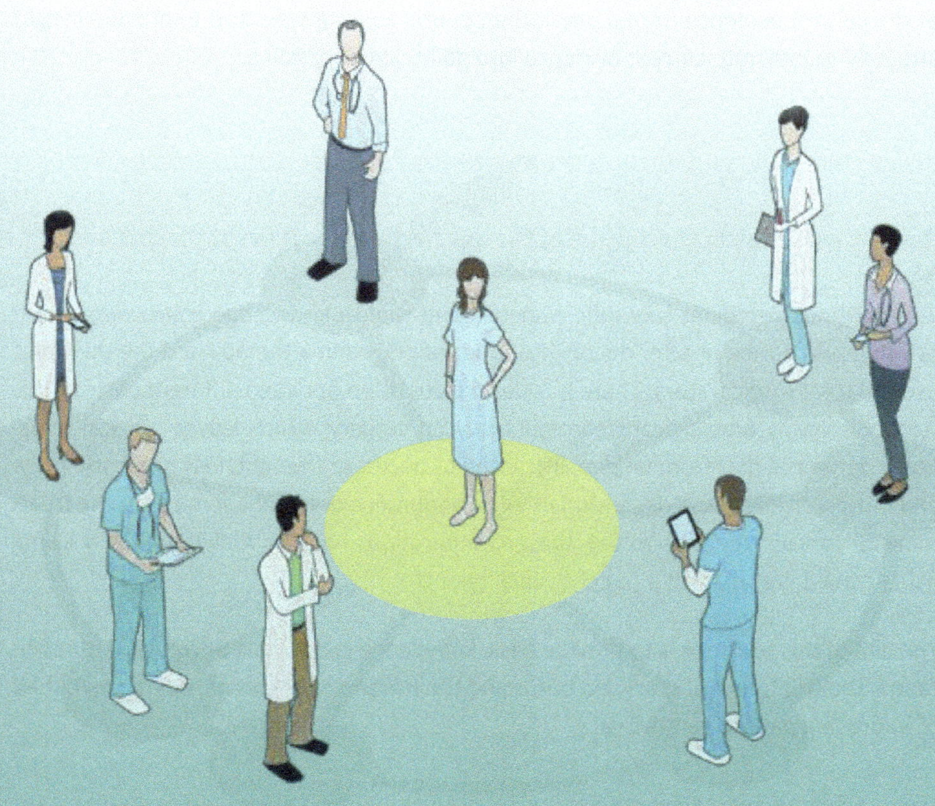

1.1   WHY DID WE WRITE THIS BOOK?

The field of oncology and lymphology is constantly expanding in knowledge. Accordingly, evidence on the physiotherapeutic modalities used is evolving as well:
- during or after the treatment of cancer;
- in oncological rehabilitation;
- in the treatment of chronic edema and breast edema;
- in the management of surgical scars.

However, there is a gap between the evidence from scientific studies and the implementation of these new insights and evidence in clinical practice, often because of a reluctance to let go of old beliefs. Therefore, this book was written to inform the reader of the current evidence from a physiotherapeutic point of view and to provide insight into how to integrate current evidence into daily clinical practice.

1.2   WHAT WILL THIS BOOK BE ABOUT?

This textbook combines scientific evidence and clinical knowledge concerning physical therapies during or after oncological treatments, edema therapy and the therapies used to treat surgical scars. There is a clear relationship between different parts of this textbook. Many oncological treatments rely on surgery, which leaves surgical scars. Many patients suffer from fatigue, increased or decreased weight, loss of muscle mass and muscle strength and decreased physical endurance or lymphedema after the treatment of cancer. Needless to say, these complications hamper Activity of Daily Living (ADL) activities and affect a patient's quality of life.

The aim of this textbook is to provide basic knowledge concerning oncological rehabilitation, the treatment of scars and burns and the treatment of chronic edema on behalf of improving patient-centred care.

1.3   FOR WHOM DID WE WRITE THIS BOOK?

Although this textbook is written by a team of authors with a strong connection to physiotherapy from both a scientific and clinical perspective, other health-care professionals will find the information in this textbook useful. Physicians will gain more insight into the conservative approaches to treating the side effects of oncological treatment, the treatment of chronic edema including breast edema and the management of surgical scars before redoing surgery to treat a scar. The textbook will also familiarize physicians with the different treatment modalities, as well as the evidence motivating the use of these modalities. As a result, physicians will be able to refer patients and prescribe physiotherapy more accurately. The information contained in this book will be of help to patient-centred care in general.

Today's care for patients, especially for patients suffering from a chronic condition, needs to start from a patient-centred view. Therefore, the information in this textbook is highly relevant to those health-care professionals (e.g., nurses, dietician, psychologists, medical suppliers) who are involved in the care of oncological patients, patients with chronic edema and patients with surgical scars. It provides them with information about the physiotherapeutic modalities and can discuss more accurately how and when other types of interventions should be implemented in the plan of care for certain patients. Our overall aim is to improve care for these types of patients.

1.4   THE EVIDENCE-BASED APPROACH

The information in this book was written based on carefully composed clinical questions using the PICOST methodology.[1] These clinical questions were answered in line with the scientific and clinical knowledge available at the moment of the writing of this textbook. After obtaining this information, the evidence was translated into the clinical reality of daily practice.

To obtain the evidence, several systematic reviews were performed. Additional information concerning the systematic reviews can be found in the online platform Sofia. Apart from the systematic reviews that were executed by the teams of the different authors, information/evidence was appraised from other guidelines, systematic reviews and meta-analysis as well as original research; all based on the 6S approach as depicted in figure 1.1.

You can find links to the International Lymphoedema Framework and the Journals at the University of Arizona on the online learning platform Sofia.

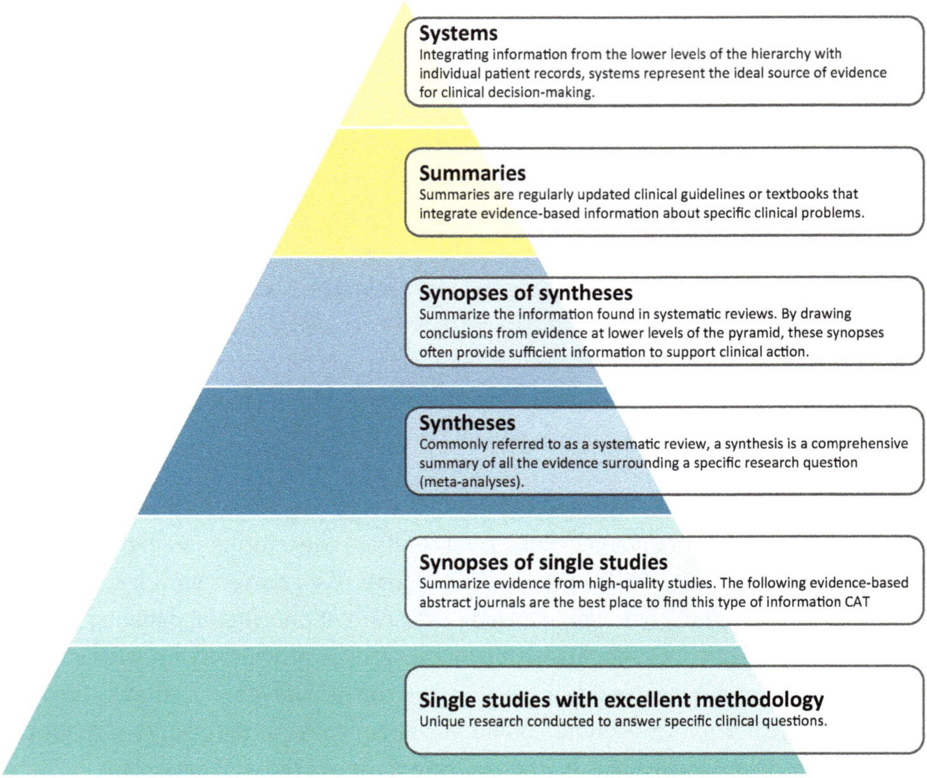
Systems
Integrating information from the lower levels of the hierarchy with individual patient records, systems represent the ideal source of evidence for clinical decision-making.
Summaries
Summaries are regularly updated clinical guidelines or textbooks that integrate evidence-based information about specific clinical problems.
Synopses of syntheses
Summarize the information found in systematic reviews. By drawing conclusions from evidence at lower levels of the pyramid, these synopses often provide sufficient information to support clinical action.
Syntheses
Commonly referred to as a systematic review, a synthesis is a comprehensive summary of all the evidence surrounding a specific research question (meta-analyses).
Synopses of single studies
Summarize evidence from high-quality studies. The following evidence-based abstract journals are the best place to find this type of information CAT
Single studies with excellent methodology
Unique research conducted to answer specific clinical questions.

Figure 1.1 The 6S pyramid for pre-appraised evidence.[2]

The clinical questions that formed the basis for retrieving the evidence used for this textbook were:

- What are the side effects (both short-term and long-term) of an oncological treatment and how can a physical treatment provide relief for these side effects?
- What are the common aspects of an oncological rehabilitation?
- Do we need to take metabolism into account when setting up an oncological rehabilitation programme?
- What are common arm and shoulder complaints that warrant a physical treatment during or after the oncological treatment of breast cancer patients in particular?
- Can preventative action be taken to avoid chronic edema formation after oncological treatments?
- What is the physical treatment of a chronic edema from a primary and secondary aetiology?
- What is the treatment of choice for treating a chronic edema in the intensive phase and maintenance phase?
- What is the current physiotherapeutic management of breast edema?
- What is the current physiotherapeutic management of surgical scars?

1.5 THE ICF MODEL AND PATIENT-CENTRED CARE

This textbook is written from a perspective that incorporates the International Classification of Functioning, Disability and Health (ICF)[3] and patient-centred care.[4]

Fortunately, for most people, functioning in daily life is something they take for granted. They can – within limits – do what they want. Yet in our care settings or in patient populations, there are people with physical and psychological problems that are so severe that they affect daily life or even make it impossible. Pain, associated with oncologic (or other) conditions, can cause sufferers to reduce their activity level significantly. Restrictions in mobility sometimes lead to not participating in sporting activities. Environmental factors, such as poor family support, colleagues who smoke or an unsuitable workplace, can adversely affect the work situation.

The ICF model (figure 1.2) was created by the World Health Organization in May 2001 to create a common language for Functioning, Disability and Health.[3]

You can find a link to the International Classification of Functioning, Disability and Health on the online learning platform Sofia.

The advantage of the ICF model is that it looks at health as a continuum and it applies to everyone. The ICF as a biopsychosocial model addresses factors at both the individual and the social level. Additionally, the ICF model focuses on both positive and negative aspects of health.[3]

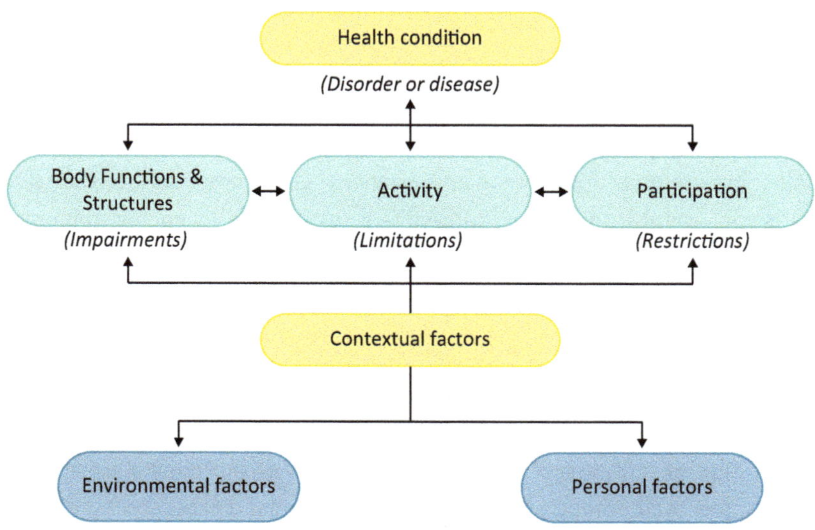

Figure 1.2   The ICF framework as described by the WHO.[3]

The ICF is a framework used around the world to describe a health condition of a patient in a broad biopsychosocial context. It applies to everyone, not just to people with functional problems. Everyone's functional health condition can be described using the ICF. It is now widely used, for instance to measure health status at the population level, in clinical and epidemiological settings to classify functional status assessment at the individual level, and to identify goal settings, treatment planning and monitoring as well as outcome measurement. The ICF describes different domains of functioning from a body, individual and societal perspective. Its core structure consists of two parts:
- functioning and disability;
- contextual factors.

1.5.1   Functioning and disability

Within functioning and disability two subcategories are recognized:
- body functions and body structures;
- activities and participation.

The **body perspective** is further divided into two components:
- The first is **body functions** and lists all physiological functions of body systems.
- The second, **body structures**, lists all anatomical parts of the body.

The individual and societal perspectives are elaborated in the component **activities** and **participation**.

1.5.2   Contextual factors

Both **environmental** and **personal factors** comprise the **contextual factors category**.

The **contextual factors** (environmental or personal factors) may affect (facilitate or inhibit) all components of functioning and disability. Environmental factors include the physical, social and attitudinal environment (e.g., profession, living environment, social support) and personal factors refer to one's attributes (e.g., age, gender, coping strategies) or internal influences on functioning.[5]

- Definition of body functions: physiological and mental (psychological) properties/functions of the human organism/body systems.
- Definition of body structures: anatomical parts of the body such as organs, limbs and their components or position, presence, shape and continuity of parts of the human body.

- Definition of activities: the execution of a task or action by an individual/components of an individual's actions.
- Definition of participation: a person's participation in society or involvement in a life situation.
- Definition of external factors: one's physical and social environment in which people live and conduct their life.
- Definition of personal factors: a person's individual background.

1.5.3   Human (dys)functioning

An individual's functioning consists of an interaction between the different components and ICF domains. There is a dynamic relationship between the ICF domains, and the interactions work in two directions, as illustrated in the figure. These components of human functioning and their problems can be represented in two ways. On the one hand, they can be used to indicate non-problematic aspects of human functioning, using the umbrella term human functioning. On the other hand, they can be used to describe disability and indicate problems, such as impairments in body function/structure, activity limitations and participation restrictions, using the umbrella term disability.

You can find a link to a practical manual on how to use the ICF on the online learning platform Sofia.

- Definition of impairments: abnormalities in or loss of functions or anatomical features.
- Definition of limitations: difficulty a person has in performing daily activities.
- Definition of participation restrictions: problems a person experiences with participating in social life.

Disability involves dysfunction at one or more of these levels: impairments in body function or structures, activity limitations and participation restrictions. Patients encountering devastating medical conditions may be confronted with long-term impairments in body structures (e.g., scars, edema) and body functioning (e.g., pain, limited mobility), activity limitations (e.g., inability to write) and participation restrictions (e.g., inability to go to school or work) during their rehabilitation. The interaction between all aspects of functioning has a dynamic character: interventions on one aspect or factor can bring about changes in other related aspects and factors. The interactions are specific and do not have a predictable one-to-one relationship. As stated earlier, the interaction takes place in both directions; the presence of functioning problems can influence a disorder or disease. It is important in the care process to collect data on these constructs independently and then to investigate possible relationships and causal links. For a complete description of (dys)functioning, all components are important. External and personal factors also influence a person's state of health and level of functioning. They can each separately or together influence functioning problems at every level.

The positive aspects and strengths within functioning can also be highlighted. The biopsychosocial vision of the ICF may make the very complex consequences of oncologic pathologies more comprehensible. The overall goal for every health-care practitioner is to recover the patients to the pre-injury state and to strive for an optimal functioning and reintegration into society with unaltered potential.

1.6   PATIENT-CENTRED CARE

Patient or client-centred care (PCC) is defined by the Institute of Medicine as follows: "Providing care that is respectful of and responsive to individual patient preferences, needs and values, and ensuring that patient values guide all clinical decisions".

In their often-cited literature review, Mead and Bower describe PCC as encompassing five conceptual dimensions:[6]
- the biopsychosocial perspective, i.e. beyond the disease state and including the psychological and social domains;
- the 'patient-as-person';
- understanding an individual's particular illness experience within his or her unique life context;
- sharing power and responsibility (an equal caregiver-patient relationship);
- the therapeutic alliance (care-giver-patient), with empathy, congruence and unconditional positive regard.

If we implement patient-centred care within the caregiver process, the use of patient-reported outcome measures (PROMs) seems imperative. PROMs are the gold standard for patient-centred care to efficiently evaluate the patient's feelings, thoughts and complaints about a clinical intervention or disease. Clinicians use PROMs to guide and audit routine care and support PCC. Many questionnaires are already part of standard intake procedures within oncologic rehabilitation. At the patient level, data can be used to monitor individual progress, investigate the effects of medical and surgical interventions and improve communication between patients and caregivers.[7] Functional outcome is often measured using PROMs. Expert consensus exists on using both generic and disease-specific Quality of Life (QoL) questionnaires to capture the full impact of a health condition.[8]

The concept of Health Related Quality of Life (HRQOL) overlaps with that of health and Quality of Life (QoL). Different definitions of these three concepts exist.[9] In this manuscript we make no explicit distinction between the different concepts and use the term QoL as an all-encompassing term to talk about HRQOL and QoL measures for the readers' convenience.

> According to the WHOQOL group (1995), QoL is defined as: "An individual's perceptions of their position in life in the context of the culture and value systems in which they live and in relation to their goals, expectations, standards and concerns. It is a broad ranging concept affected in a complex way by the person's physical health, psychological state, level of independence, social relationships and their relationship to salient features of their environment."[10]

We encourage all health-care workers to approach patients in a holistic biopsychosocial way and in a patient-centred way. These are not empty concepts but require commitment, interaction and effort from all parties involved. At regular intervals in the care process, the following questions seem important to us:
- What is my patient's wish?
- What is my patient's idea, opinion or feeling?
- How has his or her biopsychosocial functioning changed?
- How can I empower the patient as part of the (multidisciplinary) team?

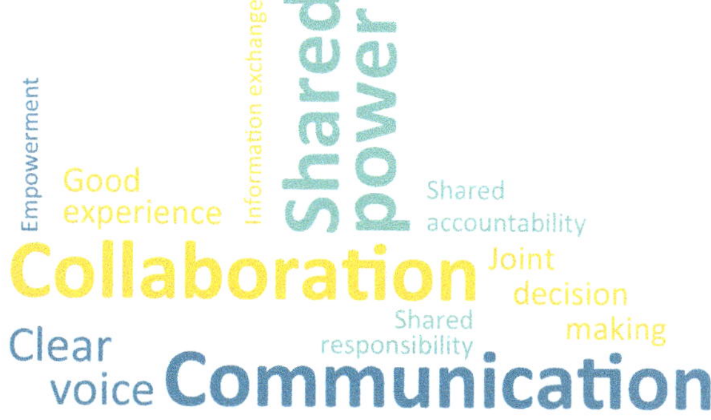

Figure 1.3   Important aspects of patient-centred care.

1.7 REFERENCES

1. Gebruers N, Meeus M. *Health Science Literacy. From research to review.* Acco; 2021.
2. DiCenso A, Bayley L, Haynes RB. ACP Journal Club. Editorial: Accessing preappraised evidence: fine-tuning the 5S model into a 6S model. Ann Intern Med. 2009;151(6):Jc3-2, jc3-3.
3. World Health O. International classification of functioning, disability and health: ICF. In. Geneva: World Health Organization; 2001.
4. Barry MJ, Edgman-Levitan S. Shared decision making--pinnacle of patient-centered care. N Engl J Med. 2012;366(9):780-781.
5. Peterson DB. International Classification of Functioning, Disability and Health: An Introduction for Rehabilitation Psychologists. Rehabilitation psychology. 2005;50(2):105-112.
6. Mead N, Bower P. Patient-centredness: a conceptual framework and review of the empirical literature. Soc Sci Med. 2000;51(7):1087-1110.
7. Meirte J, Hellemans N, Anthonissen M, et al. Benefits and Disadvantages of Electronic Patient-reported Outcome Measures: Systematic Review. JMIR Perioper Med. 2020;3(1):e15588.
8. Van Beeck EF, Larsen CF, Lyons RA, Meerding WJ, Mulder S, Essink-Bot ML. Guidelines for the conduction of follow-up studies measuring injury-related disability. J Trauma. 2007;62(2):534-550.
9. Karimi M, Brazier J. Health, Health-Related Quality of Life, and Quality of Life: What is the Difference? Pharmacoeconomics. 2016;34(7):645-649.
10. The World Health Organization Quality of Life assessment (WHOQOL): position paper from the World Health Organization. Soc Sci Med. 1995;41(10):1403-1409.

2 ONCOLOGICAL REHABILITATION

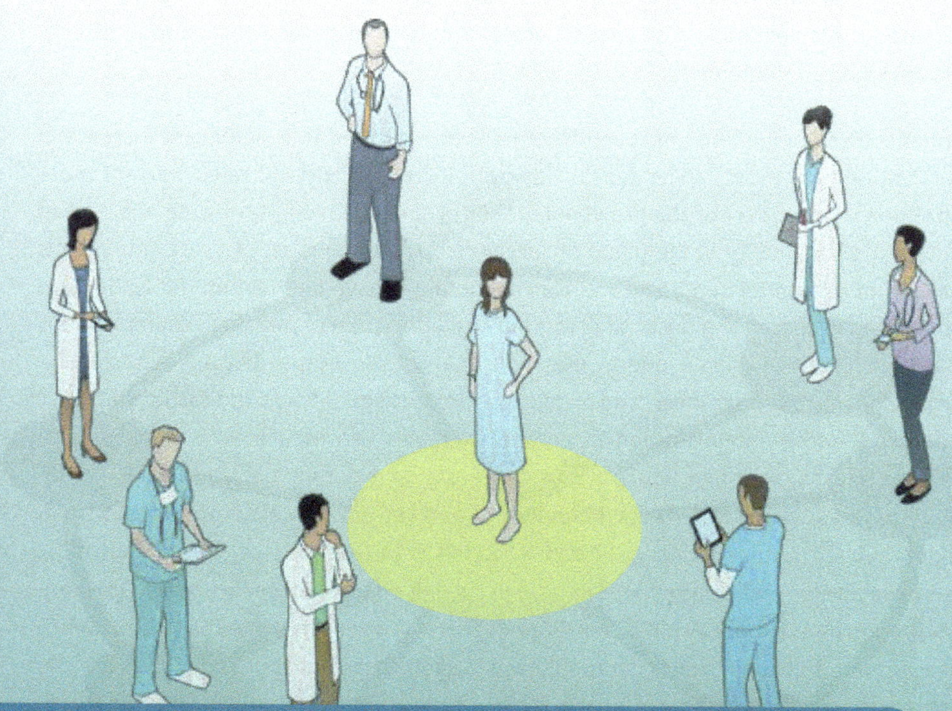

2.1 INTRODUCTION

Globally, cancer incidence and mortality rates are increasing rapidly, making cancer the second leading cause of death, with an estimated 9.6 million deaths worldwide due to cancer in 2018.[1,2] Reasons for the occurrence of cancer are complex, but both demographic changes and socio-economic factors seem to contribute.[2-4] Not all cancers are therefore completely inherited.[5] Most tumours result from external factors, interacting with daily personal habits and lifestyle manners (e.g., smoking).[1,4] Despite the growing burden, cancer survivorship has improved significantly in recent decades as a result of enhanced screening, early detection and the development of novel therapies.[2,6,7] Based on tumour type, grade, location and stage (according to the TNM classification), treatment can involve surgery, chemotherapy, radiation therapy, hormone therapy or targeted therapies that act on specific proteins in tumourigenesis (e.g., immunotherapy, angiogenesis inhibitors).[6-9]

Enhanced screening and improved treatment has resulted in a significant increase in survival rates in most cancer types. However, increased survival rates warrant more attention with respect to the growing number of short and long-term side effects that determine the quality of life (QoL) of survivors.[10] Although most of these side effects have a multifactorial aetiology, anti-cancer therapies have been identified as decisive factors in facilitating the onset of comorbid conditions.[5,11] For instance, chemotherapy is known to induce shifts in energy metabolism, most likely caused by a direct effect on intracellular protein synthesis and an altered metabolism of lipids and carbohydrates.[11] Additionally, the administration of certain therapies can induce acute after-effects, such as nausea, vomiting, mucositis or dysgeusia, and potentially lead to a lower dietary (energy) intake.[12,13] The combination of a lower energy consumption and treatment-induced metabolic changes has been found to cause cancer-related malnutrition, anorexia and/or cachexia.[12,14] These (late) occurring effects adversely impact QoL, cancer prognosis and longevity. It is therefore important to acknowledge that the presence of a tumour and concurrent treatment have a significant impact on a patient's life and are associated with long-term health (physiological, psychological and psycho-social) sequelae.[15]

There is ample evidence that factors related to lifestyle, e.g., physical activity, a healthy diet and weight management, play an important role in preventive strategies in cancer.[16] It is therefore hypothesized that cancer rehabilitation based on a healthy lifestyle might reduce treatment-related side effects and boost overall functioning in activities of daily living (ADL), consequently enhancing QoL and potentially improving cancer prognosis, survival and recurrence.[17]

2.2 CANCER- AND TREATMENT-RELATED MORBIDITIES

For many years, cancer research focused mainly on the treatment of the disease with limited attention devoted to the aftermath.[18] Due to improvements in treatment policy (patient awareness, early screening with consecutive detection) and the development of different therapies and therapeutic drugs, survivorship has increased substantially in recent decades.[19] Today, an estimated 3.4 million Europeans are newly diagnosed with cancer every year; almost 1 in 3 individuals will eventually develop a tumour during his or her lifetime.[20] Additionally, it is estimated that 50% of all patients diagnosed with cancer survive for 10 years or more.[21] The growing cancer burden in combination with increasing survival rates has led to a higher prevalence of patients and survivors with comorbidities and (chronic) health problems which require individualized follow-up to ensure the patients' QoL and functioning.[18] It is therefore important to recognize cancer- and treatment-related side effects from early on.

Side effects can arise from the disease or treatment and can be divided into two categories:
- psychological and psycho-social related morbidities;
- physiological related morbidities.

Since breast cancer is the most common type of cancer in women, it has been thoroughly investigated in scientific literature. A separate part of this chapter has therefore been devoted to breast cancer-specific morbidities (see 2.2.3 Breast cancer-related morbidities).

2.2.1 Psychological and psycho-social related morbidities

2.2.1.1 Body image and intimacy

Body image

Cancer patients undergoing treatment may lose their hair, experience changes in physical appearance due to surgery with additional (visible) scars, encounter discolouration of the skin because of irradiation, undergo unvoluntary weight changes, experience swelling of face, legs and arms (lymphedema), etc., which can lead to lower self-esteem and induce anxiety. It is important to understand how surgical interventions, radiation therapy, chemotherapeutic drugs and other treatment methods can affect a person's physical appearance in order to better prepare patients for the bodily changes that might take place.[22]

Emotional intimacy

Restoring intimacy both during and after cancer treatment can be challenging. Emotional intimacy is important, especially during treatment; many patients have already emphasized that their emotional needs were not adequately met by their caregivers. Creating time and space for maintaining an open dialogue is important in helping the patient deal with feelings of resentment, guilt, helplessness, (social) withdrawal and overall stress.[22]

Physical intimacy

Physical intimacy can be influenced by cancer treatment in many ways. Both men and women experience challenges concerning physical intimacy during and after treatment. The loss of sexual desire or difficulties with physical engagement are often described. The most common reported complications for men are erectile dysfunction and infertility. The latter is also present in women, who mention experiencing pain during sexual intercourse, as well. In both sexes, complaints go hand in hand with loss of confidence, anxiety and depression. Open communication with clinicians (e.g., psychologist, sexologist) and the partner about sexuality seems to be effective for maintaining a healthy intimate relationship.[22]

2.2.1.2   Anxiety and distress

After a cancer diagnosis, patients often encounter emotions that induce anxiety and distress (e.g., anger, fear, sadness) which are not unusual.[23,24] Anxiety and distress begin as a temporary fear or short-time worry, with feelings of restlessness, concentration difficulties and being unable to relax or control the worry or fear. In severe cases, anxiety evolves into an anxiety disorder, affecting a person's ability to lead a 'normal' life.[23] In cancer patients, tumour type does not predict the level of distress, although higher levels have been reported in patients with brain tumour and lung or pancreatic cancer.[24] The following risk factors were found to be indicative of higher levels of distress in cancer patients:[23]

- functionality problems in ADL;
- the presence of (multiple) side effects from treatment;
- problems at home;
- having unmet social and/or spiritual needs;
- cancer-related post-traumatic stress, depression and other emotional constraints;
- being female;
- being young and unable to understand the pathology and its treatment;
- having a lower level of education.

Besides its impact on the psyche, patients with anxiety report general health problems too, such as insomnia, fatigue, muscle tension, headaches and loss of appetite.[23,24] Screening for anxiety and distress when evaluating a patient's coping mechanism is important with respect to providing better (psychological) support throughout the disease trajectory.

2.2.1.3 Depression

Cancer patients experience more psychiatric unrest compared to the general population. Thirty percent of all patients with psychological distress undergo an adjustment reaction, characterized by feelings of sadness or depression within the margins of the adjustment period. Twenty percent of these patients, however, qualify for a formal psychiatric illness, of which depression is most common with an estimated prevalence between 13 and 40%.[25] Although the burden of depression in the overall cancer population is known, the majority of those suffering from depression are unrecognized and untreated. This might be the result of the fact that many patients experience 'subthreshold' symptoms without meeting the criteria for depression as described by the DSM-5 (Diagnostic and Statistical Manual of Mental Disorders, 5th version).[26] The clinical implication of depression, however, should not be underestimated. Besides its detrimental impact on the QoL, studies point out that there is a clinically significant association between depression and mortality.[25,26] Routine screening for depression should therefore be part of the multidisciplinary assessment of cancer patients and could be made a central element in patient-centred care. It has been described that treating depression improves medical outcomes, such as functional status. This raises the question of whether or not interventions on a psychological level have life-prolonging effects, but empirical evidence in this area is lacking.[25]

2.2.1.4 Social isolation

Social isolation is an important determinant that gives an indication of a patient's experience of social relationships; in this manner, it is seen as disengagement from social ties. It refers to the extent to which patients feel that the quality and quantity of their social interactions are sufficient for meeting their social needs. Indicators include feelings of loneliness, lack of social support and having little to no companionship from one's social network (e.g., community, institutional connections, family, close friends).[27,28] It is known that the impact of social isolation should not be overlooked; significant adverse effects on health outcomes and mortality have been reported in socially isolated patients. Additionally, all-cause mortality is 50% higher compared to socially integrated individuals. Moreover, factors of social isolation predict mortality comparable to those of standard clinical risk factors such as smoking, obesity and hypertension. In breast cancer patients, social isolation has been associated with an increased risk of cancer recurrence.[28]

Social isolation can be seen as a (potentially) modifiable risk factor. In that respect, it is important as clinician or caregiver to be vigilant for patient-reported symptoms such as loneliness, lack of interest, (social) withdrawal, and even poor eating and nutrition.

2.2.1.5 Return to work

Of all newly diagnosed cancer patients in Europe each year, about 50% are of working age. With better chances of survival, returning to work after cancer diagnosis and treatment has become highly important to patients, employers and, by extension, society as a whole. There are many reasons, both financial and psychological, that can motivate a cancer surviver to return to work. Studies show that work plays an important role in the formation of the survivor's identity; it builds one's self-esteem by representing capabilities and skills, and meets the need for social relationships along with the financial security it provides.[29]

Although some patients can continue working in the same manner as before the diagnosis, a large proportion of them end up with a reduced workload or even unemployment. It has also been observed that cancer survivors switch jobs more often compared to the overall healthy population. Many cancer survivors report that a lack of understanding from their work environment lies at the root of absenteeism. Additionally, a lack of understanding of employers makes survivors feel exposed and insecure about returning to work. Evidence suggests that many aspects of an employee's wellbeing are significantly determined by the employer and that they play an important role in a successful return. Clinicians should support patients in their concerns related to work and, if needed, provide information and recommendations to employers, amongst others, so that they have a better understanding of the patient's situation. This could be crucial when work needs to be adapted to the patient's reduced capacity at the time of his or her return.[29]

2.2.2 Physiological morbidities

2.2.2.1 Inflammation

Evidence regarding the determinants of cancer progression and treatment outcomes continue to be of interest to researchers and oncologists. Both tumour development and treatment can induce a variety of physiologically associated side effects.[30] Weight loss, fatigue and pain are often described as extremely debilitating and are associated with a significant deteriorating effect on QoL, response to treatment and survival.[30,31] Weight loss results from the loss of fat mass (FM) and/or fat-free mass (FFM). It can be induced by a (progressive) loss of appetite and reduced dietary intake due to nausea, dysgeusia and mucositis, all symptoms of inflammation. In recent years, the inflammatory response to the disease and/or treatment is visible in clinical practice as (an accumulation of) adverse side effects. These symptoms are important for patient assessments as they are markers of disease progression and response to treatment. Cancer- and treatment-associated inflammatory responses can be present locally, but also systemically, and are accompanied by circulating leukocytes. An acute (flare-up of) inflammation is often seen after therapy has started. However, in many cancer patients there is an ongoing chronic systemic inflammatory response.[31,32]

When inflammation lasts for too long or becomes chronic, it might lead to the development of chronic diseases, as it has been linked to a wide variety of pathologies such as Alzheimer's disease, diabetes and autoimmune diseases.[33] In cancer, the presence of circulating white blood cells was already observed in the 19th century, which was the first indication of a possible link between cancer and inflammation.[30] In general, a normal cell distinguishes itself from a tumour cell due to their difference in metabolic status, as an altered cellular metabolism is one of the main characteristics of a cancer cell. Increased metabolic fluxes and nutritional needs are required to support cell proliferation and migration to (surrounding) tissues. Next, the cell's response to hypoxia is altered because of the disbalance between the rate of tumour angiogenesis and multiplication speed of the malignant cells. Furthermore, cancer cells have deregulated apoptotic mechanisms and highly adaptive capacities for different environments, reinforcing the process of growth and metastasis. The altered tumour metabolism induces the production of, amongst others, reactive oxygen species (ROS) that add to the inflammatory milieu. These changes in (local) inflammatory status contribute to the vicious cycle that creates the tumour-indulgent environment. Inflammation therefore plays a crucial part in tumourigenesis.[30;31,33]

Cancer-associated symptoms are commonly seen as natural sequelae to the progression of the tumour. For a long time it has been known that the progression of symptoms is a harbinger of advanced disease and aggressive types of cancer.[33] A large international cohort, including 1,466 advanced cancer patients, reported a significant association between loss of appetite, pain and fatigue and C-reactive protein, an acute phase inflammatory marker.[32] Consequently, it is important to identify (systemic) inflammatory responses through clinical observation and blood serum analyses in order to provide an individual follow-up to the tumour and its response to treatment. However, some caution in the interpretation of cancer-associated morbidities in relation to disease progression is required, since it is unclear if a reduction in markers of the systemic inflammatory response, which suggests tumour reduction, will be accompanied by an improvement of these symptoms, especially during treatment.[33]

2.2.2.2 Chemotherapy-induced adverse reactions and toxicity

Chemotherapy is a frequently used modality in the treatment of cancer, often involving complex regimens of multiple drugs with narrow therapeutic index.[34,35] The overall cancer population experiences little tolerance and the use of chemotherapy makes patients highly susceptible to adverse drug reactions (ADRs); about 80% of all patients experience at least one ADR. The nature of chemotherapy, which attacks not only cancer cells but also healthy cells, sets the stage for the onset of treatment-related side effects.[36] Despite improved efficacy in battling cancer and enhanced survival offered by chemotherapy, short- and long-term morbidities remain a major source of concern.

Current drugs designed to counteract the harmful side effects of chemotherapy are often incompletely effective and do not address potential long-term morbidities. Moreover, approaches to reducing ADRs may even induce other side effects, only leading to more discomfort for patients.[35,36]

Of all acute chemotherapy-related symptoms, fatigue is the most prevalent (59-91%), followed by a decreased appetite (42-62%), nausea (28-60%), oral mucositis (17-40%) and vomiting (17-26%). Other gastro-intestinal side effects are also common and can be distressing or even fatal to patients.[37-39] Mucositis, both oral and gastro-intestinal, may affect local tissue by causing ulcers and/or pain which, in turn, can lead to anorexia, weight loss, malabsorption, anemia, fatigue and as most alarming morbidity, an increased risk of local and systemic sepsis that can cause organ damage in the long term. Adverse drug reactions can also appear weeks or even months after completion of treatment.[36] It is known that chemotherapy can affect a patient's central nervous system (CNS), giving rise to cognitive problems and memory deficits, seizures, headaches, hearing loss, etc. Besides its impact on CNS, peripheral neuropathy, myelosuppression and nephrotoxicity are also possible comorbidities that can arise. A decrease in bone mineral density might also appear after treatment, preluding osteopenia or osteoporosis.[40] One of the most life-threatening effects in the long term, however, is ROS-mediated cardiotoxicity. When severe, toxicity of the heart muscle leads to cardiac failure due to damaging of the cardiomyocytes, impairing contractile function, eventually leading to death if not treated.[41,42]

Follow-up on ADRs is necessary to support patients throughout their treatment regimen. Self-reported questionnaires on experienced symptoms are more suitable than observations by caregivers and clinicians, since the latter often underestimate the severity of complaints.[39] Moreover, specific types of chemotherapeutic agents, such as Cisplatin (alkylating agent) and Doxorubicin (anthracycline agent), are used in a wide variety of solid tumours and known to induce more ROS compared to other chemotherapeutics. Pharmacovigilance of these drugs needs to be analyzed in combination with self-reported questionnaires in order to predict the possibility of the development of ADRs and improve therapeutic strategies.[35,36,39]

2.2.2.3   Malnutrition

Malnutrition is a common, but frequently underrecognized and undertreated problem in cancer patients.[5] Malnutrition is mostly associated with undernutrition but can also result from overnutrition. An altered dietary intake, deficiencies in the absorption of specific macro- and/or micronutrients, increased nutritional losses or an increased energy expenditure (EE) because of the metabolic demand of the underlying disease can precipitate this condition. The term 'malnutrition' is used to describe a deficiency in energy balance.[12,13]

An energy balance is reached when energy consumption, meaning the total daily energy intake (TEI), equals the amount of energy spent, the total daily EE (TEE). Energy imbalances occur when intake and expenditure do not perfectly match, resulting in a change in net mass of the body's energy containing tissues, FM and FFM. This change is equal to the difference between energy intake and expenditure and can be objectified by variations in body weight (BW) and body composition ([BC]; FM or FFM).[43] A positive energy balance (TEI > TEE) promotes an increase in BW while a negative energy balance (TEI < TEE) results in weight loss.[44] The presence of cancer and/or its treatment can intensify an energy imbalance, especially undernutrition, since treatment-related side effects and changes in energy metabolism can affect a patient's normal functioning and clinical outcome.[44,45] Individual-specific nutritional support therefore plays an important role in the treatment of patients who are at risk of malnutrition in order to improve prognosis and survival.

2.2.2.4   Taste and smell alterations

Taste and smell alterations are frequently reported by cancer patients undergoing therapy and have been described as one of the most distressing side effects along with nausea, vomiting, hair loss and fatigue. They arise from either an increased or decreased sensitivity of one of the five basic taste or smell qualities (sweet, salt, bitter, sour, umami) or are the result of disturbed sensory experiences of specific nutrients, tastes or odors, due to mucositis, for example. The presence of these symptoms is primarily seen in chemotherapy and radiotherapy. Moreover, evidence is growing that other types of therapy, such as targeted- and immunotherapy, also induce changes in the perception of smell and taste regardless of cancer type. Taste and smell alterations related to chemotherapy often start early in a cycle and come and go thereafter in relation to the administration of chemotherapy. However, they do not always cease when treatment stops, and may continue for weeks (or even months). On the other hand, taste and smell alterations can also be present before therapy has started, especially in patients with head and neck cancer. This suggests that not only the treatment, but also the disease itself might induce smell- and taste-related sensory disturbances.[46,47]

The unpleasant sensations perceived when consuming food can result in a reduced dietary intake, which is alarming for the onset of malnutrition. Also, food aversion can impede social eating habits and induce mood disturbances which negatively impact social functioning and QoL.[46,47] It is therefore important to ask patients whether they are experiencing changes in smell and taste in order to identify problems in their eating (habits) and provide information and nutritional support, if necessary.

The role of fat mass and fat-free mass in cancer

The interest in understanding how measures of BC can be used to improve treatment and survival of cancer patients is growing. Body mass index (BMI; weight (kg) divided by height [m^2]) is often used as a proxy measure of total FM. According to the index, adults are classified as overweight if their BMI is between 25.0-29.9 kg/m^2 and obese if their BMI ≥ 30.0 kg/m^2.[48] Worldwide, it is estimated that 1.9 billion people are overweight, of whom more than 50% (± 650 million) are obese. Nine percent of all cancer incidences in Europe are estimated to be obesity-related, which emphasizes growing evidence that there is a correlation between BMI and an increased risk of developing certain types of cancer (e.g., colon, rectum, liver, pancreas, endometrial and post-menopausal breast cancer).[48,49]

Overweight and obesity are associated with changes in metabolic functioning, including insulin resistance, alterations in circulating growth factors and hormone levels, and systemic inflammation; all of these changes are also present in tumour development. Many of the metabolic pathways that come with these alterations are seen in cancer progression as well, suggesting that patients with BMI ≥ 25.0 have a higher risk of cancer mortality.[50] In addition, increasing BW over years is an important risk factor in the recurrence of post-menopausal breast cancer and correlates with higher mortality rates compared to patients with a normal weight. In other cancer types (e.g., leukaemia, colorectal and gastric cancer), however, BMI is not associated with a higher risk of cancer-related death and can even exhibit a protective association.[51] This has led to the 'obesity paradox', suggesting that BMI might not be the appropriate tool for investigating the relationship between cancer and BC.[49]

An explanation for the 'obesity paradox' might be that BMI is an imprecise measurement of BC. BC refers to the amount and distribution of FM (visceral, subcutaneous and intramuscular) and FFM (muscle tissue, water, bone and organs). The use of BMI can result in misclassification of the level of adipose tissue. Individuals with a normal BMI (19.0-24.9 kg/m^2) can mask excess fat tissue, while those classified as overweight do not always have the amount of FM that is associated with an increased risk of mortality.[49-51] In addition, FFM, of which muscle mass is the largest contributor, is not taken into account when BMI is calculated. Like fat tissue, skeletal muscle mass plays an important role in whole body metabolism, insulin regulation and inflammation and is an important prognostic factor of mortality. A large meta-analysis, including 7,843 breast cancer patients, found that lower muscle mass was associated with a 44% higher risk of cancer-related death.[51] The fact that overweight patients (according to BMI) have more muscle mass as well, might be an explanation for the protective association that was found in certain cancers.[12,51]

Anorexia, muscle wasting and cachexia

Two distressing comorbidities that lead to changes in BC are anorexia and muscle wasting. Anorexia is characterized by the loss of appetite. Multiple causes of anorexia in cancer patients have been reported whereby both peripheral effects, such as the release of tumour substances, dysphagia or altered gut function, and central effects as depression and pain hamper the desire to eat.[52] Loss of muscle mass is observed in muscle wasting, a condition that is present in 20-70% of the cancer population depending on method of assessment, tumour type, location and stage. This debilitating symptom can directly result from the disease, its therapy or a combination of both. Loss of muscle mass is often an occult symptom of a more severe condition (cancer cachexia).[53] Regardless of BMI, muscle wasting is considered a significant prognostic factor and is associated with cancer progression, poorer surgical outcome, higher incidence of chemotherapy related toxicity, physical impairments and shorter survival time.[12]

Both anorexia and muscle wasting are key features in the development of cancer cachexia, a multifactorial condition whereby weight loss is characterized by loss of muscle mass (thus FFM) with or without loss of FM.[12] It is present in nearly 80% of the advanced tumour stages and is the ultimate cause of death in 30% of the cancer population. Cancer cachexia is an example of malnutrition resulting from a negative energy balance (TEI < TEE). The cachectic syndrome can arise from a reduced nutrient intake or nutrient availability, secondary to anorexia or malabsorption, and an increase in metabolic demand of the tumour which contributes to muscle wasting. In addition to the metabolic perturbations, the impact of the treatment on metabolism and effects of ADR(s) might aggravate the condition. The molecular mechanisms that underlie the process of wasting have not yet been fully unraveled but available evidence suggests that increased catabolism of muscle proteins might play a prominent role, accompanied by a defective myogenesis and impaired muscle protein synthesis.[12,52,53]

The best way to manage cancer cachexia is by curing the disease. Unfortunately, this is not always possible in advanced tumour stages. The pathogenesis of cancer cachexia is multifactorial, including anorexia, metabolic disturbances, inflammation and increased muscle proteolysis. Each of these might therefore be a potential therapeutic target. While initial studies concentrated on the treatment of anorexia, the focus of therapy has shifted towards attenuating the inflammatory response and breakdown of muscle proteins.[53] In clinical settings, conservative therapies might be an important element in the support of the patient's muscle mass and physical condition. More and more studies are pointing to the long-term beneficial effects of physical exercise and resistance training during and after cancer treatment on muscle strength, cardiopulmonary function, physical functioning, QoL and fatigue.[54] It seems that the best way to prevent and treat the cachectic syndrome is multimodal, in that several aspects should be treated simultaneously.[53]

2.2.3 Breast cancer-related morbidities

For breast cancer in particular, many patients are confronted by arm and shoulder complaints. These morbidities may cause an unsatisfactory psychosocial outcome, negatively influencing activities in daily living and QoL. In recent decades, the breast cancer survival rate has increased dramatically. As such, the quality of survival, and thereby the treatment-related morbidities, have become more important. Table 2.1 provides an overview of the prevalence of the various complaints at different points in time. A differentiation is made between an axillary lymph node dissection (ALND) and the less invasive sentinel lymph node biopsy (SLNB).[55] What follows is a synopsis of complaints.

	1 week postoperative		1 month postoperative		6 months postoperative		>24 months postoperative	
	SLNB	ALND	SLNB	ALND	SLNB	ALND	SLNB	ALND
Loss of mobility	41%	86-90%	5-100%	22-100%	4-11%	2-27%	0-41%	10-80%
Pain	3-38%	31-71%	10-57%	27-79%	6-37%	2-91%	6-51%	26-79%
Loss of strength	28%	49%	-	12%	8%	15-47%	0-48%	8-60%
Numbness	7-16%	63%	4-41%	38-70%	0-43%	19-49%	5-51%	51-84%
Paresthesias	-	-	-	-	10%	19%	7-16%	19-60%

Table 2.1   Breast cancer: Prevalence of the various complaints at different points in time.

2.2.3.1 Loss of mobility

Loss of mobility in the shoulder joint after breast cancer treatment is very common and often associated with other complaints, such as: axillary web syndrome (AWS), pain, scar tissue formation, shortened pectoralis muscles, scapula alata, fibrosis of the axilla and/or chest wall, nerve damage, chronic edema, etc. In addition, fear of moving the arm postoperatively can contribute to a limited range of motion (ROM) of the shoulder. Moreover, some patients have the tendency to spare their arm. Because of this protective mannerism, a patient might adopt a different posture, which can also lead to various complaints, including loss of mobility.

In breast cancer patients, loss of mobility is mostly present during abduction and anteflexion of the shoulder. However, extension, internal and external rotation are also often limited. Research has shown that loss of mobility in the affected arm is related to loss of mobility in the contralateral arm, with the highest correlations for abduction and extension.[56] The altered posture some patients take is a possible explanation for this finding. Because of the surgery and radiotherapy that took place on the anterior chest wall, tissue damage often forces patients to adopt a protective posture. In addition, shame and fear of moving contribute to the altered posture. As a result, shortening of muscles, protraction of the shoulder and thereby shoulder girdle misalignment and scapular dyskinesias can be seen. Because of the loss of mobility in both arms, ROM should always be evaluated in both arms.

After breast cancer treatment some patients develop frozen shoulder, also called adhesive capsulitis, which results in a decrease of glenohumeral ROM and pain. The shoulder capsule, the connective tissue surrounding the glenohumeral joint, becomes inflamed and stiff, causing these symptoms.[57]

Anatomical structures on the ventral side of the chest wall can be damaged by the breast surgery and radiotherapy. This can cause scar tissue formation, fibrosis, muscle damage and inflammation. Shortening of the pectoral muscles is thus a common complaint after breast cancer treatment. Additionally, the posture can have an effect on the pectoralis muscles. As mentioned before, many patients take a protective posture due to shame, pain and anxiety, which in turn results in a protraction of the shoulder girdle. This can also explain the shortened pectoralis muscles and the subsequent loss of mobility. In this way, the protracted posture and shortened muscles perpetuate themselves.

2.2.3.2 Pain

Breast cancer can be associated with different types of pain: nociceptive pain, neuropathic pain and central sensitization. It can occur in various locations in the body and is associated with other common morbidities:

- pain in the arm: caused by AWS, chronic edema of the arm, sensitivity disturbances;
- pain in the shoulder: caused by frozen shoulder, impingement, scapula alata and other musculoskeletal dysfunctions due to altered postures and movement patterns;
- pain in the axilla: caused by AWS, sensitivity disturbances, wound healing and scar tissue formation;
- pain in the breast: caused by breast edema, wound healing, fibrosis and scar tissue formation.

Arthralgia and myalgia (joint pain and muscle pain) are commonly seen in patients who receive specific types of chemotherapy (taxanes) and/or hormone therapy (aromatase inhibitors), and is related to obesity.[58] It can occur in the elbows, hands, hips, knees and feet and is usually symmetrical. The incidence of joint pain is up to 40% in patients who received taxanes and up to 50% in those who received aromatase inhibitors.[59,60] Unfortunately, in some breast cancer patients, this serves as a reason for stopping hormone therapy, which can lead to the recurrence of breast cancer.

The postmastectomy pain syndrome (PMPS) is another type of pain seen after breast cancer treatment. It has received little attention in the literature and lacks a standardized definition or a standardized assessment tool. Its prevalence range is therefore very broad, namely 4 to 56%. The PMPS is described as a chronic neuropathic pain, caused by damage to the brachial nerve, long thoracic nerve and/or medial and lateral pectoral nerve. These nerves can get damaged during breast surgery and surgery in the axilla. Tumours in the upper outer quadrant of the breast are associated with a higher risk of developing PMPS due to the location of these nerves. In addition, the formation of scar tissue can hamper nerve function.[61]

2.2.3.3   Loss of strength

Loss of strength after breast cancer treatment is mostly seen in the shoulder abductors. However, strength in the elbow flexors and grip strength have also been shown to decrease. Several factors related to the treatment can explain this morbidity: nerve lesion after surgery, polyneuropathy after chemotherapy and/or nerve damage after radiotherapy. However, the most common cause of loss of strength in breast cancer patients is deconditioning due to disuse of the arms.

2.2.3.4   Shoulder impingement syndrome

Under normal circumstances rotator cuff tendons can move smoothly because there is enough space between the humeral head and the acromion. The surrounding bursae ensure that these structures run even smoother. However, each time the arm is elevated, there is a little bit of friction of the tendons between the humeral head and the acromion. The tendons of the rotator cuff become inflamed and in the long term they can become damaged or sometimes rupture. This leads to pain, a decrease in ROM, loss of strength and loss of function. Impingement is the biggest cause of shoulder pain, not only in breast cancer patients, but also in healthy people. Patients with impingement have difficulties with overhead activities, lifting heavy objects and lying down on the affected side.

2.2.3.5   Sensory disturbances

The intercostobrachial nerve supplies the skin of the upper half of the medial and posterior aspects of the arm and the axilla. During axillary surgery this nerve can get damaged, causing a sensory deficit in this area. Most often in the beginning after surgery, patients feel numbness in that area that can turn into a tingling feeling, called paresthesia. The sensory disturbances tend to gradually reduce, but normal sensitivity does not always return completely.[62]

2.2.3.6   Axillary web syndrome (AWS)

Axillary web syndrome (AWS) presents itself as hard strings or cords in the axilla. The strings can even extend to the forearm and/or chest or trunk. They mostly occur between 1 and 8 weeks after breast cancer surgery and resolve spontaneously within 2 to 4 months. The main symptoms are pain in the region of the strings and limited ROM.

The incidence of AWS depends on the invasiveness of the axillary surgery. After SLNB the incidence ranges between 11% and 58%. After ALND, the range is 36%-72%.[63]

AWS is poorly understood. Studies in which biopsies were taken suggest that the strings are possibly dehydrated fibrosed lymph vessels which become non-functional as a result of the dehydration; lymphatic transport through these vessels becomes therefore impossible. The precise mechanism behind the onset of AWS, however, is unclear.[64]

2.2.3.7   Scapula alata

Scapula alata or winging of the scapula is caused by a muscle deficiency of the serratus anterior muscle. This deficiency is often the result of the long thoracic nerve being injured during surgery in the axilla. In other cases, however, the nerve can get damaged by irradiation.

In patients with scapula alata, the medial border and/or inferior angle of the scapula protrudes from the back during forward flexion. In some patients, forward flexion is even too painful or impossible to execute. A positive push-up test in which the therapist places the hand of the patient against the wall with the arm 90° in forward flexion indicates a winged scapula. During the test, the patient exerts isometric force against the wall. In case of scapula alata, winging can be observed. In addition to the winging, other complaints associated with scapula alata are pain, loss of mobility – especially forward flexion and abduction of the shoulder – and loss of strength. In some patients, other muscles try to compensate for the deficiency of the serratus anterior to maintain shoulder stability. However, this can cause impingement of the rotator cuff, causing secondary pain and tendinitis. Recovery from scapula alata can usually be expected after 6 to 9 months.[55]

As for many arm and shoulder complaints after breast cancer, the incidence range for scapula alata is very broad, from 0% to 75%. One of the major contributing factors is the type of axillary surgery. The incidence of scapula alata after the more invasive ALND is much higher compared to SLNB.[65,66] Nevertheless, little research has been done with respect to scapula alata after SLNB.

2.2.3.8   Seroma

Seroma is a build-up of clear bodily fluids in places where tissue has been surgically removed. In breast cancer patients, seroma is typically present after mastectomy, breast-conserving surgery and/or lymph node removal, whereby serous fluid collection under the skin flaps or in the axillary dead space is seen.[67] Seromas tend to appear 7 to 10 days after surgery, after removal of drains. Most often, seromas resolve spontaneously over time as the body reabsorbs the fluid. This process usually takes a month. It is not necessary to treat seromas unless they are causing pain or if they are growing. When this is the case, they are most often treated by means of fine needle aspiration.

2.3 METABOLISM IN CANCER

Many of the physiological comorbidities that occur in cancer patients are the result of metabolic disturbances, either induced by the tumour itself or consequential to the negative effects of the treatment. This section focuses on how cancer and its treatment affect metabolism by altering metabolic function.

2.3.1 Molecular metabolism

2.3.1.1 Healthy cells display metabolic flexibility

Metabolism is the umbrella term for all cellular functions that either produce or consume energy in living organisms.[68,69] The set of chemical reactions, or the different metabolic pathways, that occur during cell metabolism produce energy (ATP) that is either stored or used to enable cell proliferation, division and survival. In health, metabolism strives for homeostasis and is therefore a flexible system.[70]

Metabolic flexibility can be described as the ability of an organism to respond or adapt to conditional changes in metabolic (energy) demand. Flexibility of the system requires high capabilities of energy sensing, uptake, transport and use, and is dependent on availability and requirement.[70,71] In organ tissue, the adaptability of the system is mostly seen in liver tissue, adipose tissue and muscle tissue, which govern systemic metabolic flexibility in response to a high or low energy demand (e.g., exercise vs. rest). It is the configuration of the metabolic pathways at the molecular level that ensures plasticity of the system. The process of flexibility is strictly coordinated by metabolic key enzymes and transcription factors that closely interact with mitochondria, the cell's energy (ATP) producer.[70]

The 'golden age of biochemistry' (1920s-1960s) pioneered in defining these metabolic pathways and understanding their physiological roles in nutrient (energy) utilization and energy production in living organisms. The core activity of the metabolic network is cellular respiration, a complex process involving glycolysis, conversion of pyruvate to Acetyl-Coenzyme A (AcCoA), Krebs cycle (or Tricarboxylic acid cycle (TCA cycle) and oxidative phosphorylation (OXPHOS).[69] Research on metabolic (in)flexibility has become more important since rigidity of the metabolic pathways is seen to be closely related to the development of multiple (chronic) diseases, like cancer.[70,71]

2.3.1.2 Metabolic reprogramming in cancer cells

Like any other cell in living organisms, tumour cells are entirely dependent on an adequate supply of energy in order to support cellular functioning.[72] Research on cancer metabolism is based on the principle that metabolic functioning is altered in tumour cells in order to maintain the malignant properties that are associated with the disease.

Some of these altered metabolic features have been found in multiple different tumour cells, irrespective of cancer type. Metabolic reprogramming is therefore considered a hallmark of tumourigenesis.[73]

In recent years, it has become evident that the metabolic alterations that are associated with tumourigenesis encompass all stages of tumour growth.[72,74] Cell proliferation involves several high-energy demanding anabolic reactions that produce the cell's raw materials (proteins, lipids and nucleic acids). In terms of the cell's lifespan, it has been shown that tumour cells do not only survive but also flourish as a result of meticulous selection of altered metabolic pathways that provide enough energy and metabolites, even in harsh, hypoxic and acidic conditions.[72] It seems that the reprogrammed activities support the capability of a tumour cell to adapt and survive under stressful conditions that would be harmful to most healthy cells.[72,73]

The true mechanisms behind metabolic reprogramming in tumour cells are not fully understood. At first, it was thought that mitochondria were carrying mutations that led to changes in the metabolic pathways involved in cellular respiration, making the cell functionally defective by harming its ability to achieve OXPHOS.[72,75] This theory implies that tumour cells need to adapt to the respiratory deficiency caused by these mutations. However, evidence is emerging that alterations in mitochondria are rare, and that cancer cells do not suffer from respiratory deficiencies and thus maintain the capability to carry out OXPHOS. Consequently, it can be suggested that the growing energy demand of the proliferating tumour cells is the driving force behind the metabolic reprogramming and not the mitochondrial mutations, as previously thought.[75]

Aerobic glycolysis

To meet the biosynthetic demand of cell proliferation, the import of specific nutrients from the cell's environment needs to be increased. Glucose and glutamine are two key nutrients that ensure growth and survival in mammalian cells. Besides enforcing ATP production, the catabolism of glucose and glutamine provides the cell with carbon intermediates that are used as building blocks for various macromolecules.[74,75]

Compared to healthy cells, cancer cells display a noticeable increase in glucose consumption. This phenomenon was described by the German physiologist Otto Warburg.[74] He was the first to discover one of the most frequently observed metabolic peculiarities in a great variety of tumours: the use of aerobic glycolysis over OXPHOS for the dissimilation of glucose.[74,76] In healthy cells, the process of glycolysis takes place in the cell's cytosol and degrades one molecule of glucose into two molecules of pyruvate. In absence of oxygen (O_2), pyruvate is reduced to lactate via the anaerobic glycolytic pathway resulting in two molecules of ATP. When O_2 is present, pyruvate is oxidized to yield AcCoA, that will enter the Krebs cycle. Eventually, 32 ATP molecules will be produced through OXPHOS.[76] Glycolysis is therefore a natural response to hypoxia, a situation in which O_2 is deprived, and is less efficient in producing ATP compared to OXPHOS.[75,77,78]

Warburg's discovery stated that the majority of cancer cells are dependent on a high glucose metabolism for growth and survival. Despite the high energy production through OXPHOS, cancer cells choose glycolysis even in the presence of O_2.[72,76] This phenomenon, called the Warburg effect or aerobic glycolysis, is seemingly less efficient; however, the high glycolytic turnover provides advantages for both growth and the survival of tumour cells.[72,76,78] Three possible explanations have been hypothesized for using the inefficient metabolic pathway of glycolysis over OXPHOS:[76]

- First, ATP production through glycolysis is much faster compared to OXPHOS;
- Secondly, the high glycolytic flux brings sufficient intermediates forward through the process, which are used for biosynthesis of the rapidly proliferating cells;
- Finally, accumulating levels of glycolytic intermediates in the cell's cytosol seem to have a protective effect on the cell against therapeutic drugs.

The driving force behind the increasing demand for glycolysis is hypoxia of the cancer's internal microenvironment, which is present in a wide variety of solid tumours.[72,74,79] Rapid growth of tumour cells results in rapid expansion of tumour mass, surpassing its rate of angiogenesis. This creates local ischaemic and hypoxic places inside the tumour tissue, limiting the availability of O_2 that is necessary for cell respiration. Hypoxia forces a tumour to upregulate glycolysis, while it triggers mitochondria to release ROS.[79] In low concentrations, ROS act as signaling molecules for normal processes of cell physiology, such as programmed cell death.[80,81] When ROS accumulate, oxidative stress occurs leading to ROS-mediated damage of cellular building blocks (proteins, lipids and nucleic acids), eventually leading to cellular dysfunction and apoptosis.[81] In malignant cells, however, even a moderate increase in oxidative stress has been associated with proliferation and tumour growth. This suggests that tumour cells have the capacity to adapt to oxidative stress, displaying a mutating effect of ROS on cancer cells enhancing their survival.[79]

Glutaminolysis

Next to the upregulation of glycolysis, tumour cells display an altered metabolism for glutamine. The latter is the most abundantly present amino acid in blood and the principle donor of nitrogen, which is needed for protein synthesis.[72,74,75] Mounting evidence indicates that altered glutaminolysis plays a critical role in the biosynthesis of macromolecules, the regulation of signaling pathways and maintaining redox homeostasis (via electron transport chain) which is coordinated by OXPHOS.[82] Although the mitochondrial production of ATP (through OXPHOS) decreases in cancer cells, the demand for biosynthetic precursors used for anabolic reactions, such as the synthesis of lipids and proteins, increases. A functional Krebs cycle and OXPHOS are therefore essential, implying a high need for glutamine as source of energy.[82]

Cancer cells rely on elevated glutamine metabolism in order to compensate for the increased demand of biosynthetic precursors. Higher uptake of glutamine enables ATP production through Krebs cycle and OXPHOS. The dissimilating process of glutamine, whereby specific substrates are released, provides a continuous supply of growth supporting elements.[73-75,82] Besides, glutamine is essential for the uptake of essential amino acids that are additionally used for protein and nucleotide synthesis. While mammalian cells can produce non-essential amino acids themselves, essential amino acids must be acquired from the external environment. The high requirement of malignant cells for glutamine parallels the finding of glutamine deprivation in the external tumour environment, suggesting a high influx of essential amino acids in the cancer cells. When subjected to deprivation of glutamine, neoplastic cells undergo growth arrest and cell death.[74]

In conclusion, increased glycolysis and altered glutamine metabolism contribute to the metabolic reprogramming that is seen in tumour cells. The upregulation of the glycolytic pathway, even in the presence of O_2, is called the Warburg effect (or aerobic glycolysis), and is one of the key features in a wide variety of tumours. Moreover, rapidly expanding tumours are often subjected to hypoxic conditions by surpassing angiogenesis of the micro-environment, whereby ROS are released into the cell's cytosol. Increased oxidative stress in cancer cells leads to more acidic environments, in which tumour tissue seems to thrive. This finding suggests that ROS exerts a mutating effect on cancer cells, improving their ability to adapt to their environment and enhance growth and survival. After glucose, glutamine is the second principal growth-supporting nutrient in malignant cells. Glutamine fuels the Krebs cycle and OXPHOS, a process that was first thought of as ineffective due to mitochondrial mutations. However, glutamine is used to fuel these pathways, with nitrogen and other biosynthetic precursors being released during the dissimilation process. Next, these intermediates are used as building blocks for, amongst other things, proteins and nucleic acids, which are needed for cell proliferation. Glutamine is therefore essential for tumour growth.

2.3.1.3   Chemotherapy, chemoresistance and cancer metabolism

As described above, cancer metabolism is characterized by metabolic perturbations that enhance proliferation, growth and survival of malignant cells. In order to fight tumour development, chemotherapeutic drugs are administered in the vast majority of (progressive) cancers. Chemotherapeutics are powerful chemicals that kill tumour cells by impacting one or more checkpoints in the cell's metabolism. The main goal of chemotherapy is to reduce and prevent growth and metastasis.[83] Currently, more than 200 anticancer drugs are on the market; all of these affect rapidly dividing cells and can be classified according to their action.[83,84] In general, most chemotherapeutics predominantly work on the induction of cell death.[84] Five types of cell death have been described:[84,85]

- delayed mitosis (mitotic catastrophe);
- apoptosis;
- autophagy;
- necrosis;
- senescense (permanent growth arrest inherent to ageing).

When effective, chemotherapy that focuses on cell death works on the metabolic pathways that are related to one (or more) of these types of cell death.[85]

Despite the abundant types of chemotherapeutic drugs, prognosis and outcome are far from satisfactory. Due to chemotherapy's systemic impact, not only tumour cells are attacked but also healthy cells, which is especially true in tissues displaying a high cell turnover (gastro-intestinal tract, bone marrow, skin and hair roots), giving rise to (severe) comorbidities affecting QoL and survival.[83] Despite the powerful effects of chemotherapy on tumour cells, the metabolic disturbances and adaptive capacities of the rapidly proliferating cells might counteract the impact of drug therapy on cancer metabolism, leading to the development of chemoresistance.[86]

Few reasons have been described for the development of drug resistance in tumour cells. One reason proposes that the acquisition of mutations inhibits binding to chemotherapeutics. Other theories suggest that the activity of the drug's target or multiple drug resistance transporters are upregulated. Chemoresistance can also be the result of adaptive responses occurring in the metabolic pathways downstream of the drug target, helping cancer cells withstand drug effects. The activation of DNA repair mechanisms and the upregulation of anti-apoptotic/-autophagic proteins are examples of such mechanisms.[86] Moreover, since a combination of drugs is often used, chemotherapy in itself might facilitate the development of chemoresistance by outbalancing individual drug effects.[84] Finally, intrinsic factors related to the host might also induce drug resistance. When present, chemoresistance often results in treatment failure and (eventually) death. It is important to recognize the mechanisms that are either host-related (systemically induced), tumour-related due to evolution of the disease or drug-related, and can therefore be intrinsic or acquired along the treatment trajectory.[84,87]

2.3.2 Energy expenditure

The concept of energy expenditure (EE), or, more precisely, total daily energy expenditure (TEE), has already been introduced in the previous section (see 2.2.2 Physiological related morbidities). TEE consists of different phases. Its largest component, covering

60-80% of the variances in TEE, is resting energy expenditure (REE). Another contributor is the energy that is expended in order to digest, absorb and convert food, known as diet-induced energy expenditure (DEE) (± 10% of TEE). The last component of TEE is activity-induced energy expenditure (AEE), which is the energy cost of physical activity and exercise (± 15-30% of TEE).[6,88] REE is considered to be somewhat stable over relatively short periods of time, whereas AEE and DEE can vary widely from day to day depending on performed activities and dietary consumption.[89] Therefore, REE is a more reliable parameter for research.

2.3.2.1 Resting energy expenditure and role of body composition

REE is used in clinical practice to implement nutritional interventions; it is the amount of energy that the body expends (and therefore needs) in 24 hours, in a thermoneutral, relaxed state, to maintain vital functions without losing FFM.[6,90] Ensuring normal cellular homeostasis (thus metabolism) is, along with thermoregulation, cardiac function, brain- and other nerve-related functions, one of these vital processes for life.[91] In the literature, REE is frequently used to describe a patient's metabolic state and can be assessed by the gold standard, indirect calorimetry (IC). Other methods for assessing REE are predictive equations, such as the Harris-Benedict equation (HB_{Eq}) which is, despite its limited accuracy, often used in clinical practice.[6] Measured levels of REE (REE_M) in the overall healthy population are, according to the HB_{Eq}, within 10% of the predicted REE (REE_{Pred}) and considered as normo-metabolic ($REE_M = \pm 10\% \ REE_{Pred}$).[92,93] Interestingly, a wide range of REE_M has been found in the ill population. In cancer patients, both hypometabolism ($REE_M < 90\% \ REE_{Pred}$) and hypermetabolism ($REE_M > 110\% \ REE_{Pred}$) have been found.[94] When in a hypermetabolic or hypometabolic state, the body expends respectively more and less energy than predicted. When energy requirements are not met, the metabolic state will result in weight loss (in hypermetabolism) or weight gain (in hypometabolism), seen as changes in BC, more specifically FM and FFM.[95]

BC is an important determinant of REE. In this, FFM is the largest predictor, contributing for 60-80%, while FM contributes less, approximately 30-50%. In addition, it can be said that the higher the amount of FFM the higher REE.[90,96] In general, REE is less in women compared to men, since the latter are larger in body size. What's more, men are on average heavier than women and have relatively more FFM at the same weight. An increase in BW is often the result of gaining both FM and FFM, resulting in an increase in REE. For similar reasons, REE is generally higher in those who are overweight (and obese) compared to lean people, even when matched for age, height and gender.[90,97] Changes in BC and weight have been associated with ageing, where a decrease in FFM is seen in the overall healthy elderly with controversial results for FM.[97] It is known that these changes in BC have a detrimental impact on health. A reduced QoL, immune dysfunctions, exercise intolerance and increased hospital stays have been associated with low FFM. In addition, a larger amount of FM, as seen in (sarcopenic) obesity, is related to a higher risk of metabolic disorders, cardiovascular diseases and respiratory problems.[97-99]

In clinical practice, it is important to adequately measure REE in order to implement individual-specific nutritional therapy, aiming to prevent changes in BC related to alterations in FFM and FM. The use of IC is preferred over predictive equations such as HB_{Eq}, since over- and underreporting of the true energy need have been observed in patient populations.[4]

2.3.2.2 Energy balance

An energy balance is reached when the total energy consumption throughout one day (24 h) equals the total amount of energy spent throughout the same day (TEI = TEE). It can be said that BW is an indicator for (changes in) energy balance as fluctuations in BW are seen when TEE does not equal TEI. Depletion of BW is related to a negative energy balance (TEE > TEI), while an increase is related to a positive energy balance (TEE < TEI). Besides energy intake and expenditure, energy storage is a third determinant of the energy balance and suggestive of a physiologic regulation system instead of a behavioral regulation system.[100]

The mechanisms by which the body acts to achieve and maintain an energy equilibrium are still not entirely understood. However, according to the evidence currently available, it is suggested that a complex physiological control system is required to maintain a balance between energy intake and expenditure.[101] This control system involves both afferent signals from the periphery and efferent signals from the central nervous system, with information on energy stores influencing energy intake and expenditure.[100,102] Additionally, all components of the energy balance influence one another due to external or internal shifts resulting from a positive or negative balance.[100]

Energy intake
The energy intake is characterized by three major macronutrients:
- carbohydrates;
- proteins;
- lipids.

When consumed, the net absorption of these nutrients is variable and incomplete, with faecal losses up to 10% of the gross intake. The net absorption is individual and depends on the specific foods, the way in which they were prepared and intestinal factors.[102]

In addition to food preferences and consumption, BC plays a dominant role in deciding the energy intake. FM is associated with circulating levels of leptin, a hormone that regulates satiety. As such, FM is – besides its role in energy expenditure – part of the regulatory feedback system that determines food consumption and TEI.[96,103]

Energy expenditure

Carbohydrates, lipids and proteins that have been consumed will either be stored or transformed into substrates that ultimately enter the metabolic pathways in order to produce ATP which drives biological processes. The energy that is expended reflects the macronutrients that are metabolized for physical activity, growth and many other physiologic processes.[102]

Changes in energy consumption can therefore affect energy expenditure since each fuel (nutrient) is metabolized differently. Moreover, internal processes, such as cancer metabolism, can induce changes in the metabolic pathways, energy requirements and fuel selection, eventually altering energy expenditure and storage.[102,104]

Energy storage

Energy storage reflects the net changes in metabolized carbohydrates, lipids, and proteins. Carbohydrates are mainly stored in skeletal muscle tissue and liver tissue as intracellular glycogen. The metabolism of carbohydrates into glycogen is rapid and maximal amounts are observed in the post-meal state. Muscle tissue in itself consists mostly of proteins and is its largest storage. However, lipids are the largest source of stored energy, in the form of triglycerides present in adipose tissue. Any imbalance between intake and expenditure of these macronutrients leads to a change in mass of stored energy, reflected by a change in body weight. When energy storages are addressed, a change in FM (lipids) and FFM (carbohydrates and proteins) are seen. When in health, the long-time stability of BW is often considered as net zero storage and thus energy balance.[102]

2.3.2.3 Effects of cancer and chemotherapy on energy balance in terms of resting energy expenditure

Resting energy expenditure in cancer-bearing state

In the overall cancer population, changes in REE have been seen in the tumour-bearing state. Substantial evidence supports the theory of an increase in REE, potentially resulting in weight loss due to hypermetabolism ($REE_M > 110\% REE_{Pred}$), consequential to the increase in metabolic demand due to the tumour process.[105] When the resulting energy imbalance (TEE > TEI) is not adequately met, the poor oral intake, often present in cancer patients, will accelerate weight loss enhancing malnutrition (undernutrition) and cancer cachexia.[104,106]

However, inconsistencies in REE levels have been reported across cancer types.[104] For instance, an increase in REE amongst patients with pancreatic, esophageal, gastric and lung cancer has been observed compared to healthy controls.[107] The elevation seems to be greater in lung cancer patients than in pancreatic cancer patients, although contrasting evidence exists.[108,109] Other studies report insignificant differences between patients across all advanced cancers.[109] These findings reflect the varieties in the metabolic demand of tumours, which depends on cancer type, location and stage.[104]

REE reflects the metabolic activities of body tissues and organs, and is determined by their need for energy (energy requirement). Major organs (e.g., lung, liver and skeletal muscle) are metabolically highly demanding tissues that, irrespective of health/disease, contribute to REE due to their continuous functioning, even in a resting state. It can be said that FFM is the largest contributor to REE. It is therefore valid to conclude that a loss of FFM results in a decrease in REE regardless of the circumstances.[110] However, this is not the case in cancer patients, where higher levels of REE have been measured in cancer-associated weight loss.[104]

It can be suggested that the presence of a tumour has an elevating effect on REE. The increase has been estimated to be 8-9%.[104] A plausible explanation is that the tumour production of biochemical mediators aggravates the inflammatory response, creating a tumour permissive environment stimulating cell proliferation which is enhanced by the metabolic reprogramming. The positive feedback loop of tumour growth might contribute to the increase in energy demand and the hypermetabolic state, which in turn continues to deteriorate the energy imbalance if nutritional needs are not met.[13,104,111] This theory might explain the differences in elevated levels of REE that are seen across all cancer patients.

Resting energy expenditure during and after chemotherapy

A different manifestation of REE has been observed during and after the administration of chemotherapy, with a significant decrease (- 1.5% to ± − 25%) one-month post-treatment has been found compared to pre-treatment levels in multiple cancer types (e.g., breast cancer, lung cancer and leukaemia). However, six months after finalization of the chemotherapy regimen in breast cancer, significant increases were reported compared to post-treatment, returning to pre-treatment levels.[6] The changes in REE during and after chemotherapy exhibit a U-shaped curve (figure 2.1).[4] Literature on the mechanisms causing this periodic behaviour is inconsistent. However, it is suggested that the initial decrease results from a diminished metabolic demand of the tumour in response to the given treatment.[112-114] The final increase might be attributable to the accumulative effects of chemotherapy; chemotherapeutics are known to induce complications that are related to the inflammatory process as a result of the administration of these powerful drugs.[115,116] It is clear that cancer patients undergo metabolic changes during and in the aftermath of chemotherapy. The metabolic state of a patient might fluctuate between normo-, hyper- and hypometabolism. This process is reflected by the occurring energy imbalance, seen as related changes in FM, FFM and REE.[6]

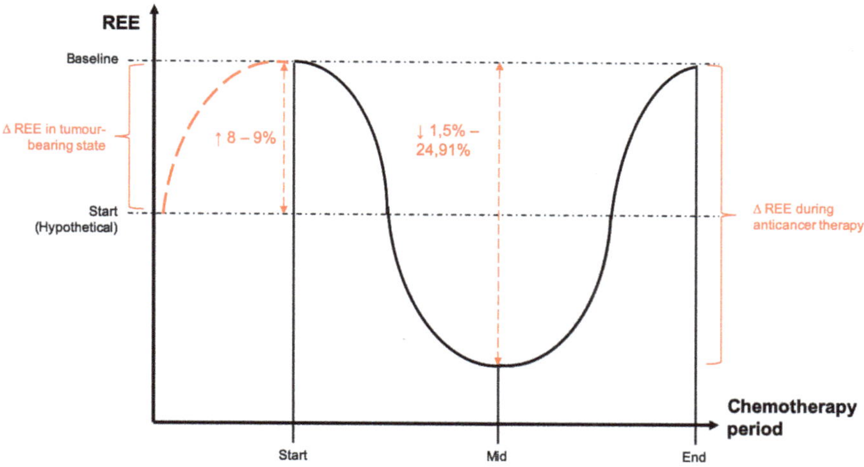

Figure 2.1   Changes in REE during and after chemotherapy: a U-shaped curve.

In clinical practice, it is important to address the metabolic fluctuations during treatment since they negatively affect cancer prognosis. Hypermetabolism in combination with a negative energy balance leads to weight loss, which can have deteriorating effects on treatment tolerance and outcome and eventually survival. Hypometabolism with a positive energy balance leads to an increase in BW. A higher BW, but more precisely a larger total amount of FM, is known to be related to the onset of certain cancer types and cancer recurrence.[117]

In conclusion, cancer has an increasing effect on REE due to the high metabolic demand of the proliferating tumour cells, irrespective of cancer type. When treated with chemotherapy, changes in REE reveal a U-shaped curve during and after completion of the treatment regimen. These changes are suggested to be a result of the positive effects on the tumour (limiting effect on tumour metabolism) and increasing systemic inflammatory response that parallels chemotherapy. Harmonizing energy intake and energy expenditure can have protective effects on the harmful conditions that can arise due to the energy imbalance. It is known that a healthy lifestyle, in terms of physical activity, nutrition and a healthy weight management, has a preventive effect on the development of cancer.[118] Addressing the (possible) energy imbalance during and after treatment might enhance treatment outcome and tumour prognosis in terms of patient survival and cancer recurrence.[119]

2.4 SUPPORTIVE STRATEGIES IN ONCOLOGICAL REHABILITATION

Early cancer research mainly focused on the development of curative therapies. In combination with early detection and increased patient awareness, improved treatment strategies have led to an increase in patient rates and a growing number of survivors.[120,121] This rising burden in cancer prevalence requires follow-up with respect to QoL, as several adverse effects of cancer and its treatment are often present.[54,121] The physiological, psychological and psychosocial sequelae are an illustration of the physical and emotional state of the patient and survivor.[120] In one out of ten patients, psychological distress is the main reason for a decreased QoL. A quarter of the patients, on the other hand, report that physical complications such as weight changes, impaired physical functioning and fatigue are the main causes of a decreased QoL.[122] It is hypothesized that conservative therapies act supportively by limiting the onset of short- and long-term morbidities. Because of this, studies on multidisciplinary oncological rehabilitation during and after treatment have gained more ground in current cancer research. Oncological rehabilitation is therefore multimodal, aiming to improve QoL by implementing psychological and psychosocial care in combination with lifestyle interventions in terms of physical activity and nutrition.[120]

2.4.1 Exercise therapy in cancer

Physical activity can be described as any bodily movement resulting from skeletal muscle activity. It can be unstructured (activities of daily life) or structured (grassroots sports, individual exercise and competitive sports) and always leads to energy expenditure.[40] Exercise therapy is an example of planned, structured and repetitive physical activity aiming to improve (physical) health.[123] Exercise is widely recognized as an effective therapy in the oncologic population. An exercise-based rehabilitation programme during or after treatment supports the patient's physical well-being and provides important benefits to the psyche. The beneficial effects on related symptoms, however, differ by type of exercise as pain reduction, for example, is found in aerobic exercise but not in resistance exercise, while fatigue improves when a combination of aerobic and resistance exercises is applied.[124] It is therefore important to adapt exercise to the needs of the individual patient (tailored approach) when implementing physical activity in the rehabilitation programme.

2.4.1.1 Therapeutic efficacy of exercise therapy

The onset of cancer and treatment related side effects can either be acute and short in duration, chronic and persisting for months or years, or late-occurring, developing months or even years after finalization of the treatment.[123] Evidence regarding the therapeutic efficacy of exercise on cancer-related health outcomes is growing but heterogeneous, as different modalities of physical activity tackle different morbidities. In 2019, the American College of Sports Medicine (ACSM) reviewed the therapeutic efficacy of physical activity for the most frequently reported cancer-related health outcomes according to the evidence found in literature (table 2.2).[125] A thorough clinical examination a priori based on patient-reported symptoms is therefore advised. In combination with standard clinical tests to assess the exercise capacity, the appropriate exercise modality can be determined and/or the rehabilitation programme adapted according to the individual need.

Strong evidence	Moderate evidence	Insufficient evidence
• Psychological distress (anxiety, depressive symptoms) • Fatigue • Health-related QoL • Lymphedema • Physical function (muscle function, cardiovascular health)	• Bone health • Sleep	• Cardiotoxicity • Cognitive function • Falls • Nausea • Pain • Sexual function • Treatment tolerance

Table 2.2   Therapeutic efficacy of physical activity as reviewed by ACSM.

Note: Moderate or insufficient evidence for specific cancer-related health-outcomes does not imply that these outcomes will not benefit in other ways from participating in physical exercise, or that patients should remain sedentary. Evidence has been graded based on current knowledge of these cancer-related morbidities as primary outcome, revealing a gap in scientific research.[125]

2.4.1.2   Exercise therapy in cancer: Development of a rehabilitation programme

It is important to keep in mind that (general) physical activity and exercise (therapy) are two different entities, as the latter is structured, planned and monitored. In the oncologic population, exercise can be prescribed in the following phases:
- pre-habilitation phase: period between cancer diagnosis and initiation of treatment;
- habilitation phase: period during cancer treatment;
- rehabilitation phase: period following finalization of treatment.

Numerous types of exercises (aerobic, resistance, strength, weight and impact, balance and flexibility and relaxation) can be prescribed and combined, depending on the patient and his/her disease or treatment-related morbidities.[123] For exercise therapy, it is known that one size does not fit all. A well-designed exercise prescription is therefore warranted. Cancer care, however, is dynamic, and previously designed exercise regimens may not be tenable throughout the whole rehabilitation. It is therefore important to regularly follow up on clinical symptoms.[126] Table 2.3 shows the different types of exercises and their influence on cancer- and treatment-related side effects.

	Aerobic exercise	Resistance exercise	Strength exercise	Weight & Impact exercise	Balance exercise	Flexibility & Relaxation exercise
Psychological and psycho-social morbidities						
Pain	x					
Fatigue	x	x	x			x
Sleep disorders	x					x
Depression, Anxiety	x					
QoL	x	x	x			x
Self-esteem		x				
Physiological morbidities						
Bone loss and Disease		x		x		
Muscle and fat mass imbalance	x		x			
Cachexia	x	x				
Peripheral neuropathy			x			
Lymphedema	x	x	x	x		

Adapted from Ellahham.[123]

Table 2.3 Different types of exercises and their influence on cancer- and treatment-related side effects.

Pre-exercise evaluations

The concurrent cancer- and treatment-related side effects with sometimes pre-existing health conditions often deter individuals from participating in physical exercise programmes. In addition, environmental and motivational constraints and safety concerns are barriers that prevent patients from engaging in exercise therapy. It is therefore important to determine the individual's risk for adverse cardiovascular events related to physical activity by evaluating the prior level of function, exercise habits, lifestyle manners, pre-existing morbidities and environmental situation. Promoting exercise therapy requires a pragmatic approach, with the patient being repeatedly screened for clinically meaningful changes from baseline assessments.[126]

Current literature suggests that exercise has a low incidence of adverse events related to physical activity in cancer patients. Therefore, exercise therapy appears to be relatively safe, although the characteristics of the tumour and given treatment may not be ignored, as certain cancer types and therapeutic drugs are more harmful than others. A clinical decision tree for assessing the risk of adverse events during physical activity has been developed based on best available knowledge and clinical experience (figure 2.2). This decision tree can be used to help clinicians evaluate their patient as high, intermediate or low risk for adverse events and recommend patient-specific exercise requirements.[127] If uncertainties arise, referral to the oncologist for risk assessment is advised.

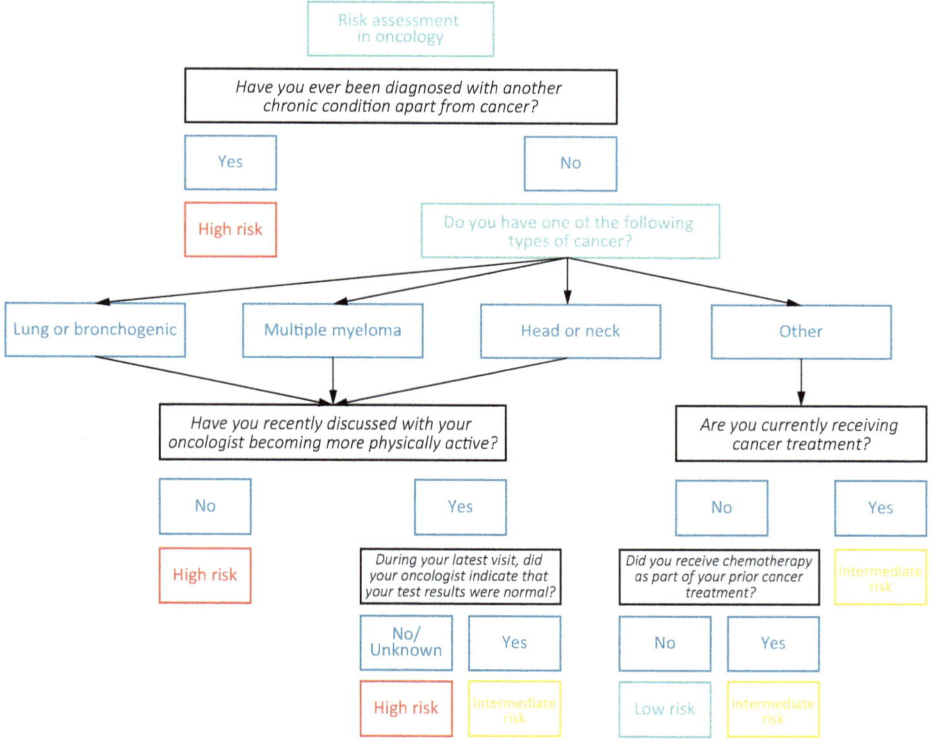

Figure 2.2 Clinical decision tree for assessing the risk of adverse events during physical activity in cancer patients.

Exercise-related clinical evaluations

The evaluation of all the different components related to physical fitness (cardiorespiratory fitness, muscle strength and endurance, flexibility and body composition) should be the cornerstone in assessing one's exercise capacity, physical functioning and health.[125]

Accurate exercise tests are therefore crucial and can reveal physical limitations that affect performance. Individual exercise tests are reliable methods for designing a patient-tailored exercise programme. In the oncologic population, some recommendations for testing must be kept in mind (table 2.4).[125] In addition, it is of utmost importance to follow up on the individual physical progress (or decline), whereby frequent re-testing throughout the rehabilitation programme is advised. Methods for testing the exercise capacity can be maximal (by cardiopulmonary exercise testing [CPET] or a steep ramp test [SRT]) or submaximal (by a six-minute walk test [6-MWT] or Astrand test).[128]

Standard exercise testing methods are generally appropriate for patients with cancer who do not require pre-exercise medical evaluation or who have been medically cleared for exercise with the following considerations:

1. Be aware of the health history, comorbid chronic diseases and health conditions, and any general exercise contra-indications before commencing health-related fitness assessments or designing the exercise prescription.
2. Be familiar with the most common toxicities associated with cancer treatments, including increased risk for fractures and cardiovascular events, along with neuropathies or musculoskeletal morbidities related to specific types of treatment.
3. Health-related fitness assessments may be valuable for evaluating the degree to which components of fitness have been affected by cancer-related fatigue or other commonly experienced symptoms that impact function.
4. There is no evidence that the level of medical supervision required for symptom-limited or maximal cardiopulmonary exercise testing needs to be different for patients with cancer than for other populations.
5. The evidence-based literature indicates 1-Repetition maximum (1RM) testing is safe among survivors of breast and prostate cancer without bony metastases.
6. Among patients with bony metastases or known or suspected osteoporosis, routine assessments of muscle strength and/or endurance involving musculature that attaches to and/or acts on a skeletal site that contains bone lesions should be avoided. Medical clearance by a physician may be mandatory.
7. Older survivors and/or survivors treated with neurotoxic chemotherapy (typical for breast, colon, lung, ovarian cancers) may especially benefit from a standard assessment of balance and mobility to assess fall risk.
8. Pre-exercise screening for cardiovascular disease is advised (figure 2.2).

Adapted from Campbell et al.[125]

Table 2.4 Cancer-specific recommendations for exercise testing.

- Cardiopulmonary exercise testing (CPET): The most direct method of assessing one's aerobic fitness is through a CPET evaluation, which is recommended in the exercise guidelines for people with cancer. Peak oxygen uptake (O_{2peak}) is the best indicator of the individual cardiopulmonary fitness and can only be measured by CPET through continuous analysis of gas exchange. O_{2peak} reflects the ability of the cardiopulmonary system to deliver oxygen to the skeletal muscles and their efficiency to utilize oxygen during maximal exertion. In addition, O_{2peak} is a strong predictor of survival in the general population. This makes CPET an excellent diagnostic tool before the start of a rehabilitation programme. Besides monitoring gas exchange, CPET also provides information on cardiac function (by electrocardiography) and workload during rest, submaximal and maximal exertion. These results can reveal possible limitations in cardiac, pulmonary, or skeletal muscle function, resulting in a more complete image of the individual's physical performance. When using a CPET protocol, exercise programmes can be tailored based on a percentage of O_{2peak}, a percentage of maximal heart rate (HR_{max}) or HR at the anaerobic treshold.[129]

- Steep ramp test (SRT): In daily clinical practice, direct measurements of O_{2peak} by CPET is expensive in terms of skilled staff and equipment. Moreover, the maximal exercise test puts a serious burden on the patient as far as exercise time is concerned. In this respect, the steep ramp test (SRT) can be a safe and valid alternative. The SRT determines the maximum short-exercise capacity by monitoring maximum workload and HR_{Max}. It is an incremental test that is short in duration but with a fast increase in workload. Since it does not involve respiratory gas analysis, the total cost is limited. The SRT has been shown to be suitable for assessing aerobic fitness in the adult cancer population, as it is highly correlated with CPET results and has a good test-retest reliability. The SRT can therefore be used for prescribing training loads and monitoring training progress.[128]

- Six-minute walk test (6-MWT) or Astrand test: The 6-MWT or Astrand test are submaximal exercise tests that are easy to perform and often readily available. Submaximal tests assess the functional capacity, with the maximal exercise performance being deduced from HR at submaximal workload. However, clinicians should be careful when interpreting field tests as they are not designed to determine peak performance and/or maximal load. In clinical populations, submaximal tests might therefore not serve as valid alternative to CPET or as the method of choice for developing exercise programmes. However, in combination with a maximal exercise test at baseline, field tests can serve as a quick and easy method for an intermediate follow-up between two consecutive CPETs or SRTs.[130]

The gold standard for evaluating muscular strength is dynamometry (for upper and lower extremities) or, in clinical practice, the 1 Repetition Maximum (1-RM) test. This test assesses the maximum load that a person (or muscle group) can possibly lift for one repetition. The most widely used exercises to determine 1-RM addressing multiple large muscle groups are bench press and leg press for the upper and lower body, respectively. Other exercises that focus on specific muscles or muscle groups are also possible. Muscle endurance, on the other hand, can be measured by using a fixed percentage of 1-RM or a fixed weight, whereby the total number of repetitions is evaluated. Norm values exist for both muscle strength and muscle endurance. However, these norm values are not always applicable in the oncologic population as external factors (e.g., treatment, fatigue) can influence the outcome. Therefore, it is recommended to use the 1-RM and muscle endurance test only for the individual exercise prescription and performance follow-up.[131]

Evaluation of flexibility

Flexibility is, along with aerobic exercise capacity, muscle power and muscle endurance, an important component of physical fitness and used to describe the range of motion (ROM) of a single, or series, of joints. Within sport, many activities are based on the ROM of the lower extremity, where high performance levels are correlated with a high degree of flexibility in specific joints. Consequently, tight connective tissue around the joints and/or short muscles might make an athlete susceptible to possible muscle strain or joint injuries. Flexibility is therefore a parameter of muscle health. In cancer patients, muscle weakness due to reduced protein synthesis and muscle degradation may occur, leading to a decreased functional performance, decreased flexibility and reduced mobility, all affecting the QoL. To support muscle health, it is important to implement field tests that evaluate flexibility in the pre-exercise assessment. A common test used for the measurement of lower limb flexibility is the classic (or modified) sit-and-reach test, while the shoulder flex test is indicative of upper limb flexibility.[132]

Evaluation of body composition

There is a growing interest from the cancer community in understanding how measures of body composition can be used to support cancer treatment and survivorship. Recent observational studies have indicated that both the distribution of adipose tissue (fat mass (FM)) and muscle mass (MM) are risk factors for clinical outcomes, as an increase in chemotherapy-related toxicity and postoperative complications are frequently seen. This underscores the need for evaluating body composition, as cancer patients are often older adults who might already experience age-related changes in body composition that might be further exacerbated by the disease and/or treatment.

It is hypothesized that addressing body composition in cancer rehabilitation can offer additional benefits to patients both during and after treatment.[48]

- **Body mass index (BMI):** The body mass index (BMI) can be calculated by assessing body weight (kg) and dividing it by body height (m) squared. The BMI can be used to interpret weight status:
  - < 18.5 = underweight;
  - 18.5-24.9 = normal or healthy weight;
  - 25.0-29.9 = overweight;
  - > 30.0 = obese.

  However, the usability of BMI in clinical populations is under debate, as it tends to overestimate total FM in people with a high amount of MM and tends to underestimate FM in elderly who often display muscle atrophy. Clinicians should therefore be careful when interpreting BMI, as it is not the appropriate tool for a complete analysis of body composition in patients with excess adiposity or poor muscle health. Besides, BMI provides no information regarding the distribution of adipose tissue. For that reason, additional evaluations are advised.

- **Abdominal obesity:** The distribution of adipose tissue can be investigated by the presence of abdominal obesity, and can be calculated by dividing waist circumference (cm) by hip circumference (cm) (i.e. waist-to-hip ratio [WHR]). The World Health Organization defines abdominal obesity as a waist circumference of more than 102 cm in men and 99 cm in women. The presence of abdominal obesity has been linked to the onset of many metabolic diseases and, in some types of cancer, tumour development as well. Follow-up of WHR can therefore provide information on body fat distribution and might provide a rationale for weight-related interventions.

- **Percentage of fat mass:** The percentage of total FM (%FM) can be derived from skinfold measurement. Four skinfolds (biceps, triceps, subscapular, suprailiac) are measured and %FM (from total body weight) is then calculated by using the equation of Durnin and Womersley.[133] The correlation between skinfold measurements with calculation of %FM according to Durnin and Womersley and dual-energy X-ray absorptiometry (DEXA, gold standard) has been extensively investigated. However, for patients at risk of malnutrition or negative outcomes related to body weight or body composition, evaluation by the gold standard should be considered.

Exercise prescription in cancer: Frequency, intensity, duration and type

The benefits of exercise on physical health in the cancer-free population are widely documented. Consequently, a key consideration in many study trials implementing physical activity has been whether or not cancer patients and survivors can endure exercise training doses that are known or hypothesized to have positive effects on physical fitness and in turn on disease or treatment-related outcomes. To date, research has shown that patients and survivors effectively respond to physical activity with improved muscle strength and endurance, cardiovascular fitness and body composition. However, individuals might respond differently to a given exercise stimulus which might be due to the specific cancer treatment, disease type or stadium or demographic factors (e.g., age). Moreover, exercise tolerance of both patients and survivors can vary from training to training. Monitoring physical functioning and understanding the interactions with external stimuli can help to adapt the exercise programme to the individual's needs.

Exercise programmes can consist of various combinations of aerobic and resistance exercises based on frequency (number of times per week), duration (number of minutes per session) and intensity. The intensity of an exercise or exercise training is related to the energy that is expended, which depends on how hard the body must work during that specific exercise. The exercise intensity can either be objectified by measuring oxygen uptake (by gas analysis) or HR during activity, calculated by metabolic equivalents (METS), or subjectively reported with a self-reported estimate of effort (Rate of Perceived Exertion [RPE]) on a scale of 1-10. Intensities can vary between the following, with concordant changes in HR:

- sedentary-low (efforts < 1-3 times of the energy expended in rest);
- moderate (efforts between 3-6 times the energy expended in rest);
- vigorous-high (efforts > 6 times the energy expended in rest).

An overview of the different intensities and related objective and subjective measures is displayed in table 2.5.

Intensity category	Objective measures	Subjective measures
Sedentary	< 1.6 METS < 40% HR_{max} < 20% O_{2peak}	RPE < 1/10
Low	1.6 – 3 METS 40 – 55% HR_{max} 20 – 40% O_{2peak}	RPE = 1-2/10
Moderate	3 – 6 METS 55 – 70% HR_{max} 40 – 60% O_{2peak}	RPE = 3-4/10
Vigorous	6 – 9 METS 70 – 90% HR_{max} 60 – 85% O_{2peak}	RPE = 5-6/10
High	≥ 9 METS ≥ 90% HR_{max} ≥ 85% O_{2peak}	RPE ≥ 7/10

Adapted from Norton et al.[134]

Table 2.5 Overview of intensities and related objective/subjective measures.

The following recommendations have been made regarding the specific exercise prescription in cancer:[125]

- Cancer patients undergoing active treatment or after completion of treatment can safely participate in exercise rehabilitation programmes, of at least 8 weeks, though 12 weeks or more is preferred, at moderate intensities as recommended by the ACSM:
  - Aerobic exercise:
    - frequency: 3-5 times per week;
    - intensity: moderate;
    - duration: 150 min in total; at least 30 min per session;
    - warm-up and cool-down included.
  - Resistance exercise:
    - frequency: 2-3 times per week;
    - intensity: at least 60% of 1 Repetition Maximum; 8-10 muscle groups;
    - repetitions: 8-10 repetitions; 2 sets;
    - warm-up and cool-down included.
- Moderate exercise is expected to improve the QoL, muscle function and aerobic fitness of cancer patients. Depending on the type of exercise, different outcomes can be expected (table 2.6).

Aerobic exercise	Resistance exercise	Combination exercise
• Reduced anxiety • Fewer depressive symptoms • Less fatigue • Better QoL • Improved perceived physical function	• Less fatigue • Better QoL • No risk of exacerbating lymphedema • Improved perceived physical function	• Reduced anxiety • Fewer depressive symptoms • Less fatigue • Better QoL • Improved perceived physical function

Adapted from Campbell et al.[125]

Table 2.6 Expected outcomes of exercise rehabilitation.

- It is recommended for cancer patients to train in a group setting or a supervised setting.
- It is recommended for cancer patients to implement exercise at moderate intensities on an ongoing basis in their lifes in order to maintain the beneficial effects on QoL, muscle function and aerobic fitness in the long term.

Accessibility to exercise rehabilitation

- **Patient-reported barriers:** It is not easy to convince cancer patients and survivors to participate in exercise rehabilitation programmes. Barriers to joining can be classified according to disease-specific limitations (e.g., fatigue, pain), socio-economic barriers (e.g., lack of time, financial difficulties) and individual barriers (e.g., social withdrawal, lack of motivation, decreased self-esteem). Fear of pain or fatigue is reported most due to the belief that cancer management requires rest instead of exercise. It is the clinician's task to help the patient to overcome these barriers.[125]

- Motivation can be created through patient education. Counselling and motivational interviewing with physical therapists and physicians can encourage patients to enrol in a rehabilitation programme. It is important that expectations and attitudes toward exercising are made clear to the patient before the start of the programme. The principles of exercise training should be explained to and understood by the patient. At least the first sessions should be supervised by a physical therapist (or trainer) to ensure the correct performance of exercises, though supervision throughout the programme is ideal. The physical therapist appears to play a fundamental role in the adherence of patients and survivors to a programme, underscoring the need for educated practitioners.

- The monitoring of physical performance (e.g., HR, workload) and symptoms (e.g., fatigue, pain) before, during and after the training sessions and activities outside the rehabilitation setting can also help to educate the patient and increase motivation.

- Ideally, exercise therapy should be implemented at the time of diagnosis, with the aim being to reduce morbidities resulting from the disease and treatment. When offering physical activity at the beginning of the treatment, it is hypothesized that patients will have the physical capacity to enrol in rehabilitation programmes after treatment. If patients are already used to physical activity, maintenance of the activity status can be expected.

- It can be said that adherence to exercise increases as the patient keeps moving, regardless of the motivation at the beginning of the programme. However, 50% of all patients enrolled in a rehabilitation programme stop before the end. It is therefore essential to create an individual-tailored programme based on the individual exercise capacity, as this increases feasibility. Social support from caregivers or exercising with companions can also improve adherence.[125]

2.4.2 Nutrition therapy in cancer

In addition to physical activity, individual nutritional interventions are also valuable in patient-centred care, as the nutritional state is often impaired. Nausea and vomiting, symptoms of occult toxicities of the gastro-intestinal tract, can lead to reduced food intake. When severe or occurring over a prolonged time, the nutritional state may deteriorate, which can cause interruption of the treatment, worsening of QoL and deterioration of the clinical prognosis. Given this scenario, adopting a balanced diet (according to the individual energy needs) is important on behalf of preventing nutritional deficiencies and improving the nutritional state and QoL.[135]

2.4.2.1 Therapeutic efficacy of nutrition therapy

Malnutrition in terms of weight loss is a common phenomenon in the oncologic population, with an incidence rate of 40-80% depending on tumour type, stage, location, treatment and method of assessment. In cancer, especially cancer of the gastrointestinal tract, a poor QoL, high postoperative morbidity and mortality and low treatment tolerance have been correlated with a deteriorated nutritional state.[136] Weight loss can be related to either physiological abnormalities induced by the tumour (e.g., vomiting, obstruction, diarrhea, malabsorption of nutrients), the host's response to the tumour (e.g., altered energy metabolism, anorexia), or side effects resulting from the anticancer treatment. Progressive weight loss, general physical weakness and cachexia are responsible for up to 20% of cancer-related casualties. Cancer cachexia appears as final outcome of the disturbances in the absorption of nutrients, alterations in appetite, taste and total energy intake, changes in hormone balance or energy metabolism, and altered immune response related to the disease. Weight loss has a decreasing effect on the innate immune response to tumour cells and the ability of the system to oppose infections, which increases susceptibility to future complications.[137]

In contrast, malnutrition in terms of weight gain also occurs during chemotherapy, especially in breast cancer patients. Possible risk factors for an increase in body weight are radiotherapy, hormone therapy and hormone receptor status, menopausal state, metastasis in neighboring lymph nodes, age and BMI. The differences in weight during chemotherapy are related to food intake, type of chemotherapeutic drugs and medication. However, it is difficult to pinpoint the true causes of weight gain, as it can also be explained by the presence of common side effects of chemotherapy. For instance, fatigue potentially leads to a reduction in habitual physical activity, while disturbances in energy metabolism consequential to the administration of chemotherapy might cause alterations in energy expenditure.[138]

It has been been found that well-nourished patients experience better therapeutic tolerance, especially against chemotherapy, less toxicities related to the treatment, better response to treatment and adherence to treatment schedules, lower infection rates and decreased risk of early death.[137]

2.4.2.2 Nutrition therapy in cancer: Development of dietary interventions

Nutritional support must be tailored (in collaboration with the dietician) to the individual patient and requires adequate evaluation and follow-up. In doing so, the clinical assessment of the nutritional state, the identification of a specific therapeutic drug and the treatment planning and expected outcome must be considered.

Clinical evaluation of the nutritional state

Risk stratification

All oncologic patients should be screened for the risk of nutritional deterioration at an early stage. It is therefore recommended to regularly evaluate the nutritional intake, changes in body weight and BMI either directly or by means of validated nutritional screening tools. Some qualitative tools for risk detection that can be used depending on the clinical setting are:[139,140]

- outpatient clinic: Malnutrition Universal Screening Tool (MUST);
- inpatient clinic: Nutrition Risk Screening 2002 (NRS-2002);
- elderly: Mini Nutritional Assessment – Short Form (MNA).

Nutritional assessment

If abnormal screening is present, an objective and quantitative assessment of the dietary intake and nutrition impact symptoms, physical performance, body composition (FM and FFM) and degree of systemic inflammation is recommended. The Patient Generated Subjective Global Assessment tool (PG-SGA) is a valid and reliable tool that combines semi-quantitative and qualitative data and can be used in both the ambulatory and acute care setting to identify energy intake and related symptoms. Physical performance can either be determined by CPET or rated using scales (ECOG Performance status, Karnofsky Performance status), dynamometry or 1-RM measurement, or gait speed. In malnourished patients, it is strongly advised to assess muscle mass by DEXA scan or computed tomography scan (CT) at lumbar level 3. Finally, the degree of systemic inflammation can be estimated by serum analysis of C-reactive protein (CRP) and albumin.[139,140]

Assessment of energy requirements

Various methods have been developed to determine the energy requirements (energy expenditure, EE) in clinical practice. For example, the predictive Harris-Benedict Equation (HB_{Eq}), is based on anthropometric variables, which makes it easy to apply in daily care.[141] Although the validity of predictive equations has been shown in the overall healthy population in absence of any disease or intervention (e.g., medication), EE, especially resting energy expenditure (REE), is often underestimated in acute hospitalized patients (see 2.3.2.3 Effects of cancer and chemotherapy on energy balance in terms of resting energy expenditure).[142] An accurate analysis of (R)EE in the individual patient, especially malnourished patients or ones at risk, is therefore of fundamental importance.

The gold standard for measuring EE is indirect calorimetry (IC). IC assesses EE by measuring real-time oxygen consumption (O_2) and carbon dioxide production (CO_2). Their ratio (provides the respiratory quotient (RQ), which varies depending on oxidized nutrients (proteins, fats or carbohydrates) at that moment. The largest component of the total daily energy requirements (total daily energy expenditure, TEE) is REE, which is therefore often measured in clinical (and research) settings. The ratio of measured levels of REE (REE_M) to predicted levels of REE (REE_{Pred}) provides information on one's metabolic state, which can either be hypermetabolic (REE_M > 10% REE_{Pred}), hypometabolic (REE_M < 10% REE_{Pred}) or normometabolic (REE_M = ± 10% REE_{Pred}) (see 2.3.2.1 Resting energy expenditure and role of body composition).[143]

Information on body weight and body composition, the nutritional state, an accurate analysis of the energy requirements (especially REE) and oxidized nutrients (by RQ) and a determination of the metabolic state (normo-, hyper-, or hypometabolic) provide the rationale for a patient-tailored implementation of dietary interventions that can support the patient through his/her disease trajectory.

Development of nutrition therapy

Nutrition therapy during cancer

It is known that chronic malnutrition results from an insufficient diet. A stable nutritional state is reached when the total daily energy intake (TEI) meets the total daily EE (TEE). The latter is the sum of resting EE (REE), activity-induced EE (AEE) and diet-induced EE (DEE). In cancer patients, REE as determined by IC has been reported to have increased, decreased or unchanged in relation to non-cancer bearing controls. These variations in REE are present regardless of weight changes characterized by changes in body composition (FM and/or FFM) (see 2.3.2.3 Effects of cancer and chemotherapy on energy balance in terms of resting energy expenditure). However, when TEE is considered, lower values have been noticed compared to healthy controls, which appears to be the result of a reduction in physical activity. In absence of valid assessment methods (IC), it can be hypothesized that nutrition therapy can be initiated under the assumption that TEE is similar to healthy controls.[140] However, when IC is available, accurate assessment of REE is advised. It has been found that dietary interventions based on IC show a more adequate intake of calories and proteins compared to subjects with prediction-based interventions. IC is therefore strongly recommended in malnourished patient populations and patients at risk of malnourishment in order to maximize the benefits of nutrition therapy.[143]

The following strong recommendations (with low to strong consensus) regarding nutrition therapy in the oncologic population have been made by the European Society of Parenteral and Enteral Nutrition (ESPEN):[140]

- If not measured individually by indirect calorimetry, the TEE can be assumed to be similar to healthy controls, generally ranging between 25-30 kcal/kg/day;
- The intake of proteins should be above 1g/kg/day and, if possible, up to 1.5 g/kg/day;
- The supplementation of vitamins and minerals should not exceed the daily allowance, except in the presence of specific deficiencies;

- In cancer patients who are losing weight and experiencing insulin resistance, dietary interventions should aim to reduce the glycemic load. This should involve increasing the ratio of energy resulting from fats to energy resulting from carbohydrates;
- Nutritional interventions should aim to increase oral intake in patients who are malnourished (or at risk of malnutrition) but able to eat. If patients are unable to eat, enteral nutrition must be considered over parenteral nutrition;
- It is not recommended to use dietary provisions restricting energy intake in the malnourished or patients at risk of malnutrition;
- If oral food intake has been limited or decreased severely for a longer period, it is recommended to slowly increase nutrition (oral, enteral or parenteral) over several days. In doing so, clinicians should remain vigilant for symptoms of refeeding syndrome related to metabolic disturbances;
- Together with nutritional interventions, it is strongly recommended to maintain or increase the level of physical activity, aiming to support physical functioning, muscle mass and the metabolic pathways. It has been proven that individual-tailored exercise therapy is well-tolerated and safe at different stages of cancer; even in advanced stages, as long as patients are willing to participate in an activity-based rehabilitation programme.

Nutrition therapy after cancer

Extended survivorship is a measure of treatment success. However, a substantial proportion of the cancer survivors will experience cancer recurrence, grow second tumours or develop other metabolic conditions such as cardiovascular disease (CVD) or obesity. This can partially be explained by lifestyle behaviour. Although some survivors might have adopted a healthier lifestyle, many maintain habits akin to those of the general population – a population characterized by overweight or obesity, inactivity and high-fat diets with low consumption of fibre, vegetables and fruits. As cancer survivors often display higher rates of comorbidities, such as fatigue, food intolerances, digestive disorders, weight disturbances and aberrations in energy metabolism affecting the energy balance, nutrition therapy also has a place in post-treatment, patient-centred care. Nutrition therapy can provide a basis for changes in lifestyle behaviour that promote general health and consequently limit the onset of comorbidities and/or cancer recurrence.[144]

2.4.3 Lifestyle in terms of physical activity and nutrition: Implications for primary and secondary cancer prevention

Improved cancer treatments and methods for tumour detection are not likely to eradicate cancer and the burden of cancer completely. Evidence is accumulating that primary prevention of tumour development and prevention of cancer recurrence rely on the same principles of a healthy lifestyle. Expert reports and consensus statements of leading cancer societies all emphasize the importance of weight control, physical activity and a healthy diet in primary and secondary prevention of cancer.[145]

The following guidelines have been developed by the American Cancer Society (ACS) regarding nutrition and physical activity for primary and secondary cancer prevention and should be kept in mind in patient-centred oncological rehabilitation (table 2.7).

Achieve and maintain a healthy weight throughout life	<ul><li>Be as lean as possible throughout life without being underweight.</li><li>Avoid excess weight gain at all ages. For those who are currently overweight or obese, losing even a small amount of weight has health benefits and is a good place to start.</li><li>Engage in regular physical activity and limit consumption of high-calorie foods and beverages as key strategies for maintaining a healthy weight.</li></ul>
Adopt a physically active lifestyle	<ul><li>Adults should engage in at least 150min of moderate intensity or 75min of vigorous intensity activity each week, or an equivalent combination preferably spread throughout the week.</li><li>Children and adolescents should engage in at least 1hr of moderate or vigorous intensity activity each day, with vigorous intensity activity occurring at least 3 days/week.</li><li>Limit sedentary behavior.</li><li>Doing some physical activity above usual activities can have many health benefits.</li></ul>
Consume a healthy diet, with an emphasis on plant foods	<ul><li>Choose foods and beverages in amounts that help achieve and maintain a healthy weight.</li><li>Limit consumption of processed meat and red meat.</li><li>Eat at least 2.5 cups of vegetables and fruits each day.</li><li>Choose whole grains instead of refined grain products.</li><li>Limit alcohol consumption: No more than one drink/day for women or two drinks/day for men.</li></ul>

Adapted from Kushi et al.[145]

Table 2.7 ACS Recommendations for individual lifestyle choices regarding physical activity and nutrition.

What the physiotherapist, physician and (social) nurse need to know:
- Comorbid conditions can arise from both the tumour and treatment, and affect all aspects of the patients' QoL.
- Some psychological and psycho-social related morbidities are related to an increased risk of mortality.
- (Energy) metabolism is disturbed in cancer patients and requires individual follow-up.
- Exercise therapy and nutrition therapy during and after treatment have beneficial effects on adherence to treatment, response to treatment, prognosis, survivorship and QoL.
- Exercise therapy and nutrition therapy should be tailored to the individual patient.
- The physiotherapist can play an important role in oncological rehabilitation and close cooperation can add to better patient support.
- Specific recommendations for both exercise therapy and nutrition therapy can help educate the patient.
- Healthy lifestyle interventions related to exercise therapy and nutrition are beneficial in both the primary and secondary prevention of cancer.

What the dietician needs to know:
- Nutrition therapy should be tailored to the patient based on REE assessment with gold standard (indirect calorimetry).
- The energy need during and after cancer treatment varies and should be regularly assessed.
- Nutrition therapy both during and after cancer treatment is advised.
- Healthy lifestyle interventions related to exercise therapy and nutrition are beneficial in both the primary and secondary prevention of cancer.

What the psychologist needs to know:
- Some psychological and psycho-social related morbidities are related to an increased risk of mortality.
- Exercise therapy has beneficial effects on the psyche (collaboration).

English terms	Nomina anatomica
Glenohumeral joint	Art. glenohumeralis
Intercostobrachial nerve	N. intercostobrachialis
Long thoracic nerve	N. thoracicus longus
Medial pectoral nerve	N. pectoralis medialis
Lateral pectoral nerve	N. pectoralis lateralis

English terms	Nomina anatomica
Humeral head	Caput humeri
Serratus anterior muscle	M. serratus anterior
Medial border of the scapula	Margo medialis scapulae
Inferior angle of the scapula	Angulus inferior scapulae

2.5 REFERENCES

1. World Health Organization (WHO). Cancer. Published 2018. https://www.who.int/news-room/fact-sheets/detail/cancer
2. Bray F, Ferlay J, Soerjomataram I, Siegel RL, Torre LA, Jemal A. Global cancer statistics 2018: GLOBOCAN estimates of incidence and mortality worldwide for 36 cancers in 185 countries. Ca Cancer J Clin. 2018;68(6):394-424.
3. Torre LA, Siegel RL, Ward EM, Jemal A. Global Cancer Incidence and Mortality Rates and Trends – An update. Cancer Epidemiol Biomarkers Prev. 2016;25(1):16-27.
4. Van Soom T, Tjalma W, El Bakkali S, Verbelen H, Gebruers N, van Breda E. Perspective: Towards personalised metabolic coaching in cancer. Facts Views Vis Obgyn. 2018;10(3):125-130.
5. Tan SY, Poh BK, Nadrah MH, Jannah NA, Rahman J, Ismail MN. Nutritional status and dietary intake of children with acute leukaemia during induction or consolidation chemotherapy. J Hum Nutr Diet. 2013;26(1):23-33.
6. Van Soom T, El Bakkali S, Gebruers N, Verbelen H, Tjalma W, van Breda E. The effects of chemotherapy on energy metabolic aspects in cancer patients; A systematic review. Clin Nutr. Published online 2019.
7. Urruticoechea A, Alemany R, Balart J, Villaneuva A, Vinals F, Capella G. Recent advances in cancer therapy: an overview. Curr Pharm Des. 2010;16(1):3-10.
8. Gebski V, Burmeister B, Smithers BM, Foo K, Zalcberg J, Simes J. Survival benefits from neo-adjuvant chemoradiotherapy or chemotherapy in oesophageal carcinoma: a meta-analysis. Lancet oncol. 2007;8(3):226-234.
9. Baudino T. Targeted Cancer Therapy: The next generation of cancer treatment. Curr Drug Discov Technol. 2015;12:3-20.
10. Burke S, Wurz A, Bradshaw A, Saunders S, West MA, Brunet J. Physical activity and quality of life in cancer survivors: A meta-synthesis of qualitative research. Cancers (Basel). 2017;9((5)).
11. Sinno MH, Coquerel Q, Boukhettala N, Coeffier M, Gallas S, Terashi M. Chemotherapy induced anorexia is accompanied by activation of brain pathways signaling dehydration. Physiol Behav. 2010;101(5):639-648.
12. Nicolini A, Ferrari P, Masoni MC, Fini M, Pagani S, Giampietro O. Malnutrition, anorexia and cachexia in cancer patients: A mini-review on pathogenesis and treatment. Biomed Pharmacother. 2013;67(8):807-817.
13. Fearon K, Arends J, Baracos V. Understanding the mechanisms and treatment options in cancer cachexia. Nat Rev Clin Oncol. 2013;10(2):90-99.
14. Purcell SA, Eliott SA, Baracos VE, Chu QS, Prado CM. Key determinants of energy expenditure in cancer and implications for clinical practice. Eur J Clin Nutr. 2016;70(11):1230-1238.
15. Demark-Wahnefried W, Jones LW. Promoting a helathy lifestyle among cancer survivors. Hematol Oncol Clin North Am. 2009;22(2):319-342.
16. Rock CL, Doyle C, Demark-Wahnefried W, et al. Nutrition and physical activity guidelines for cancer survivors. Ca Cancer J Clin. Published online 2012.
17. Denlinger CS, Ligibel JA, Are M, et al. NCCN guidelines insights: Survivorship, Version 1.2016. J Natl Compr Canc Netw. 2016;14:715-724.

18. Lagergren P, Schandl A, Aaronson N, et al. Cancer survivorship: An integral part of Europe's research agenda. Mol Oncol. 2019;13(3):624-635.

19. Malvezzi M, Bertuccio P, Rosso T, et al. European cancer mortality predictions for the year 2015: does lung cancer have the highest death rate in EU women? Ann Oncol. 2015;26(4):779-786.

20. Ferlay J, Steliarova-Foucher E, Lortet-Tieulent J, et al. Cancer incidence and mortality patterns in Europe: estimates for 40 countries in 2012. Eur J Cancer. 2013;49(6):1374-1403.

21. Allemani C, Matsuda T, Di Carlo V, et al. Global surveillance of trends in cancer survival 2000-14 (CONCORD-3): analysis of individual records for 37 513 025 patients diagnosed with one of 18 cancers from 322 population-based registries in 71 countries. Lancet. 2018;391(10125):1023-1075.

22. Bates G, Taub R, West H. Intimacy, body image and cancer. JAMA Oncol. Published online 2016.

23. National cancer institute. Adjustment to Cancer: Anxiety and distress (PDQ(r))-patient version. https://www.cancer.gov/about-cancer/coping/feelings/anxiety-distress-pdq

24. Bates G, Mostel J, Hesdorffer M. Cancer-Related anxiety. JAMA Oncol. 2017;3(7).

25. Pinquart M, Duberstein P. Depression and cancer mortality: A meta-analysis. Psychol Med. 2010;40(11):1797-1810.

26. Lloyd-Williams M. Depression – The hidden symptom in advanced cancer. J R Soc Med. 2003;96(12).

27. Zhu V, Lenert L, Bunnell B, Obeid J, Jefferson M, Hughes Halbert C. Automatically identifying social isolation from clinical narratives for patients with prostate cancer. BMC Med Inform Decis Mak. 2019;19(43).

28. Pantell M, Rehkopf D, Jutte D, Syme L, Balmes J, Adler N. Social Isolation: A predictor of mortality comparable to traditional clinical risk factors. Am J Public Health. 2013;103(11):2056-2062.

29. de Rijk A, Amir Z, Cohen M, et al. The challenge of return to work in workers with cancer: employer priorities despite variation in social policies related to work and health. J Cancer Surviv. 2020;14:188-199.

30. Roxburgh C, McMillan D. Cancer and systemic inflammation: Treat the tumour and treat the host. Br J Cancer. 2014;(110):1409-1412.

31. Singh N, Baby D, Prasad Rajguru J, Patil P, Thakkannavar S, Bhojaraj Pujari V. Inflammation and Cancer. Ann Afr Med. 2019;18(3):121-126.

32. Laird B, Fayers P, Fearon K, Kaasa S, Fallon M, Klepstad P. The systemic inflammatory response and it relationship to pain and other symptoms in advanced cancer. Oncologist. 2013;18(9):1050-1055.

33. Neagu M, Constantin C, Popescu J, et al. Inflammation and metabolism in cancer cell – mitochondria key player. Front Oncol. 2019;9:348.

34. McTiernan A, Jinks R, Sydes M, et al. Presence of chemotherapy-induced toxicity predicts improved survival in patients with localised extremity osteosarcoma treated with doxorubicin and cisplatin: A report from the European Osteosarcoma Intergroup. Eur J Cancer. 2012;48(5):703-712.

35. Toale K, Johnson T, Ma M. Chemotherapy-induced toxicities. In: Oncologic Emergency Medicine. Springer; 2016:381-406.

36. Chopra D, Rehan H, Sharma V, Mishra R. Chemotherapy-induced adverse drug reactions in oncology patients: A prospective observational survey. Indian J Med Paediatr Oncol. 2016;37(1):42-46.

37. Nurgali K, Jagoe R, Abalo R. Editorial: Adverse effects of cancer chemotherapy: Anything new to improve tolerance and reduce sequelae? Front Pharmacol.

38. Pearce A, Haas M, Viney R, et al. Incidence and severity of self-reported chemotherapy side effects in routine care: A prospective cohort study. PLoS One. 2017;12(10).

39. Wang T, Samuel J, Brown M, et al. Routine surveillance of chemotherapy toxicities in cancer patients using the patient-reported outcomes version of the common terminology criteria for advere events (PRO-CTCAE). Oncol Ther. 2018;(6):189-201.

40. Ferioli M, Zauli G, Martelli A, et al. Impact of physical exercise in cancer survivors during and after antineoplastic treatments. Oncotarget. 2018;9(17):14005-14034.

41. Yang M, Moon C. Neurotoxicity of cancer chemotherapy. Neural Regen Res. 2013;8(17):1606-1614.

42. Angsutararux P, Luanpitpong S, Issaragrisil S. Chemotherapy-Induced cardiotoxicity: Overview of the roles of oxidative stress. Oxid Med Cell Longev. Published online 2018.

43. Saunders J, Smith T. Malnutrition: causes and consequences. Clin Med. 2010;10(6):624-627.

44. Ahmed N, Choe Y, Mustad V, et al. The impact of malnutrtion on survival and healthcare utilization in Medicare beneficiaries with diabetes: a retrospective cohort analysis. BMJ Open Diabetes Res Care. Published online 2017.

45. Lam Y, Ravussin E. Analysis of energy metabolism in humans: A review of methodologies. Mol Metab. Published online 2016.

46. Zabernigg A, Gamper E-M, Giesinger J, et al. Taste alterations in cancer patients receiving chemotherapy: A neglected side effect? Oncologist. 2010;15(8):913-920.

47. Belqaid K, Tishelman C, Orrevall Y, Mansson-Brahme E, Bernhardson B-M. Dealing with taste and smell alterations – A qualitative study of people treated for lung cancer. PLoS One. 2018;13(1).

48. Brown J, Cespedes Feliciano E, Caan B. The evolution of body composition in oncology-epidemiology, clinical trials, and the future of patient care: Facts and numbers. J Cachexia Sarcopeni. 2018;9(7):1200-1208.

49. Caan B, Cespedes Feliciano E, Kroenke C. The importance of body composition in explaining the overweight paradox in cancer. Cancer Res. 2018;78(8):1906-1912.

50. Lauby-Secretan B, Scoccianti C, Loomis D, Grosse Y, Bianchini F, Straif K. Body fatness and cancer – Viewpoint of the IARC working group. N Engl J Med. 2016;375(8):794-798.

51. Protani M, Coory M, Martin J. Effect of obesity on survival of women with breast cancer: systematic review and meta-analysis. Breast cancer res treat. 2010;123(3):627-635.

52. Ezeoke C, Morley J. Pathophysiology of anorexia in the cancer cachexia syndrome. J Cachexia Sarcopeni. 2015;6(4):287-302.

53. Pin F, Barreto R, Couch M, Bonetto A, O'Connell T. Cachexia induced by cancer and chemotherapy yield distinct perturbations to energy metabolism. J Cachexia Sarcopeni. 2019;(10):140-154.

54. De Backer IC, Vreugdenhil G, Nijziel MR, Kester AD, van Breda E, Schep G. Long-term follow-up after cancer rehabilitation using high-intensity resistance training: persistent improvement of physical performance and quality of life. Br J Cancer. 2008;(99):30-36.

55. Adriaenssens N, De Ridder M, Lievens P, et al. Scapula alata in early breast cancer patients enrolled in a randomized clinical trial of post-surgery short-course image-guided radiotherapy. World J Surg Oncol. 2012;10.

56. Verbelen H, Gebruers N, Eeckhout F-M, Verlinden K, Tjalma W. Shoulder and arm morbidity in sentinel node-negative breast cancer patients: a systematic review. 2014;144(1):21-33.

57. Yang S, Park D, Ahn S, et al. Prevalence and risk factors of adhesive capsulitis of the shoulder after breast cancer treatment. Support Care Cancer. 2017;25(4):1317-1322.

58. Din O, Dodwell D, Wakefield R, Coleman R. Aromatase inhibitor-induced arthralgia in early breast cancer: what do we know and how can we find out more? Breast Cancer Res Treat. 2010;120(3):528-538.

59. Winters-Stone K, Schwartz A, Hayes S, Fabian C, Campbell K. A Prospective Model of Care for Breast Cancer Rehabilitation : Bone Health and Arthralgias. Cancer. 2012;118(S8):2288-2299.

60. Galantino M, Desai K, Greene L, Demichele A, Tompkins Stricker C, Mao J. Impact of Yoga on Functional Outcomes in Breast Cancer Survivors With Aromatase Inhibitor – Associated Arthralgias. Integr Cancer Ther. 2012;11(4):313-320.

61. Alves Nogueiro Fabro E, Bergmann A, Do Amaral E Silva B, et al. Post-mastectomy pain syndrome: Incidence and risks. Breast. 2012;21(3):321-325.

62. Wijayasinghe N, Andersen K, Kehlet H. Neural blockade for persistent pain after breast cancer surgery. Reg Anesth Pain Med. 2014;39(4):272-278.

63. Koehler L, Haddad T, Hunter D, Tuttle T. Axillary web syndrome following breast cancer surgery: symptoms, complications, and management strategies. Breast Cancer: Targets and Therapy. 2018;2019(11):13-19.

64. Moskovitz A, Anderson B, Yeung R, Byrd D, Lawton T, Moe R. Axillary web syndrome after axillary dissection. Am J Surg. 2001;181(5):434-439.

65. Nevola Taixeira L, Lohsiriwat V, Schorr M, et al. Incidence, predictive factors, and prognosis for winged scapula in breast cancer patients after axillary dissection. Support Care Cancer. 2014;22(6):1611-1617.

66. Langer I, Guller U, Berclaz G, et al. Morbidity of sentinel lymph node biopsy (SLN) alone versus SLN and completion axillary lymph node dissection after breast cancer surgery: a prospective Swiss multicenter study on 659 patients. Ann Surg. 2007;245(3):452-461.

67. Srivastava V, Basu S, Shukla V. Seroma formation after breast cancer surgery: What we have learned in the last two decades. J Breast Cancer. 2012;15(4):373-380.

68. Metallo C, Vander Heiden M. Understanding metabolic regulation and its influence on cell physiology. Mol Cell. 2013;49(3):388-398.

69. DeBerardinis R, Thompson C. Cellular metabolism and disease: What do metabolic outliers teach us? Cell. 2012;148(6):1132-1144.

70. Smith R, Soeters M, Wüst R, Houtkooper R. Metabolic flexibility as an adaptation to energy resources and requirements in health and disease. Endocr Rev. 2018;39(4):489-517.

71. Goodpaster B, Sparks L. Metabolic flexibility in health and disease. Cell Metab. 2017;25(5):1027-1036.

72. Dias Amoêdo N, Perez Valencia J, Figueiredo Rodrigues M, Galina A, Rumjanek F. How does the metabolism of tumour cells differ from that of normal cells. Biosci Rep. 2013;33(6).

73. DeBerardinis R, Chandel N. Fundamentals of cancer metabolism. Sci Adv. 2016;2(5).

74. Pavlova N, Thompson C. The emerging hallmarks of cancer metabolism. Cell Metab. 2016;23(1):27-47.

75. Gentric G, Mieulet V, Mechta-Grigoriou F. Heterogeneity in cancer metabolism: New concepts in an old field.

76. Yu L, Chen X, Sun X, Wang L, Chen S. The glycolytic switch in tumours: How many players are involved? J Cancer. 2017;8(17):3430-3440.

77. Cooper G. The Cell: A Molecular Approach 2nd Edition. Sunderland; 2000.

78. Zheng J. Energy metabolism of cancer: Glycolysis versus oxidative phosphorylation (review). Oncol Lett. 2012;4(6):1151-1157.

79. Shi D-Y, Xie F-Z, Stern J, Liu Y, Liu S-L. The role of cellular oxidative stress in regulating glycolysis energy metabolism in hepatoma cells. Mol Cancer. 2009;(8):32.

80. Tauffenberger A, Fiumelli H, Almustafa S, Magistretti P. Lactate and pyruvate promote oxidative stress resistance through hormetic ROS signaling. Cell Death Dis. 2019;10(653).

81. Ray P, Huang B-W, Tsuji Y. Reactive oxygen species (ROS) homeostasis and redox regulation in cellular signaling. 2012;24(5):981-990.

82. Jin L, Alesi G, Kang S. Glutaminolysis as a target for cancer therapy. Oncogene. 2016;35(28):3619-3625.

83. Akhdar H, Legendre C, Aninant C, More F. Anticancer Drug Metabolism: Chemotherapy resistance and new therapeutic approaches. In: Topics on Drug Metabolism. InTech; 2012.

84. Guo W, Tan H-Y, Chen F, Wang N, Feng Y. Targeting cancer metabolism to resensitize chemotherapy: Potential development of cancer chemosensitizers from traditional chinese medicines. Cancers (Basel). 2020;12(2):404.

85. Ricci M, Zong W-X. Chemotherapeutic approaches for targeting cell death pathways. Oncologist. 2011;11(4):342-357.

86. Zaal E, Berkers C. The influence of metabolism on drug response in cancer. Front Oncol. 2018;8(500).

87. Alfarouk K, Stock C-M, Taylor S, et al. Resistance to cancer chemotherapy: Failure in drug response from ADME to P-gp. Cancer Cell Int. 2015;15(71).

88. Heydenreich J, Kayser B, Schutz Y, Melzer K. Total energy expenditure, energy intake, and body composition in endurance athletes across the training season: A systematic review. Sports Med Open. 2017;3(8).

89. Anthanont P, Jensen M. Does basal metabolic rate predict weight gain? 2016;104(4):959-963.

90. Westerterp K. Control of energy expenditure in humans. In: Endotext.; 2000.

91. Pelley J. Nutrition. In: Elseviers's Integrated Review Biochemistry (Second Edition).; 2012.

92. Douglas CC, Lawrence JC, Bush NC, Oster RA, Gower BA, Darnell BE. Ability of the Harris Benedict formula to predict energy requirements differs with weight history and ethnicity. Nutr Res. 2007;27(4):194-199.

93. Boothby WM. Summary of the basal metabolism data on 8,614 subjects with especial reference to the normal standards for the estimation of the basal metabolic rate. J Biol Chem. 1922;54:783-803.

94. Knox LS, Crosby LO, Feurer ID, Buzby GP, Mullen JL. Energy expenditure in malnourished cancer patients. Ann Surg. 1983;197(2):152-162.

95. van den Berg MM, Winkel RM, de Kruif JT, van Laarhoven HW, Visser M, de Vries JH. Weight change during chemotherapy in breast cancer patients: a meta-analysis. BMC cancer. 2017;17(1):259.

96. Müller M, Bosy-Westphal A, Later W, Haas V, Heller M. Functional body composition: Insights into the regulation of energy metabolism and some clinical applications. Eur J Clin Nutr. 2009;(63):1045-1056.

97. Genton L, Graf C, Karsegard V, Kyle U, Pichard C. Low fat-free mass as a marker of mortality in community-dwelling healthy elderly subjects. Age Ageing. 2013;42(1):33-39.

98. Janssen I. Morbidity and mortality risk associated with an overweight BMI in older men and women. Obesity. 2007;15:1827-1840.

99. Pichard C, Kyle U, Morabia A, Perrier A, Vermeulen B, Unger P. Nutritional assessment: Lean body mass depletion at hospital admission is associated with an increased length of stay. Am J Clin Nutr. 2004;79:613-618.

100. Hill J, Wyatt H, Peters J. Energy balance and obesity. Circulation. 2012;126(1):126-132.

101. Sandoval D, Cota D, Seeley R. The integrative role of CNS fuel-sensing mechanisms in energy balance and glucose regulation. Ann Rev Physiology. 2008;(70):513-535.

102. Hall K, Heymsfield S, Kemnitz J, Klein S, Schoeller D, Speakman J. Energy balance and its components: Implications for body weight regulation. Am J Clin Nutr. 95(4):989-994.

103. Fujita Y, Katsuyasu K, Ohara K, Nakamura H, Iki M. Leptin mediates the relationship between fat mass and blood pressure. Medicine. 2019;98(12).

104. Nguyen T, Batterham M, Edwards C. Comparison of resting energy expenditure between cancer subjects and healthy controls: a meta-analysis. Nutr Cancer. 2016;68(3):374-387.

105. Baumgartner RN, Heymsfield SB, Roche AF. Human body composition and the epidemiology of chronic disease. Obes Res. 1995;3.

106. Fredrix E, Soeters P, Wouters E, Deerenberg I, von Meyenfeldt M, Saris W. Effect of different tumour types on resting energy expenditure. Cancer res. 1991;51(22):6138-6141.

107. Cao D-X, Wu G-H, Zhang B, et al. Resting energy expenditure and body composition in patients with newly detected cancer. Clin Nutr. 2010;29:72-77.

108. Fearon K, Hansell D, Preston T, et al. Influence of whole body protein turnover rate on resting energy expenditure in patients with cancer. Cancer Res. 1988;48:2590-2595.

109. Trutschnigg B, Kilgour R, Morais J, et al. Metabolic, nutritional and inflammatory characteristics in elderly women with advanced cancer. J Geriatr Oncol. 2013;4:183-189.

110. Nielsen S, Hensrud DD, Romanski S, Levine JA, Burguera B, Jensen MD. Body composition and resting energy expenditure in humans: role of fat, fat-free mass and extracellular fluid. Int J Obes. 2000;(24):1153-1157.

111. Falconer J, Fearon K, Plester C, Ross J, Carter D. Cytokines, the acute-phase response, and resting energy expenditure in cachectic patients with pancreatic cancer. Ann Surg. 1994;219(4):325-331.

112. Jebb SA, Osborne RJ, Dixon AK, Beehen NM, Elia M. Measurements of resting energy expenditure and body composition before and after treatment of small cell lung cancer. Ann Oncol. 1994;(5):915-919.

113. Galati PC, Chiarello PG, Simoes BP. Variation of resting energy expenditure after the first chemotherapy cycle in acute leukemia patients. Nutr Cancer. 2016;68(1):86-93.

114. Lerebours E, Tilly H, Rimbert A, Delarue J, Piguet H, Colin R. Change in energy and protein status during chemotherapy in patients with acute leukemia. Cancer. 1988;61(12):2412-2417.

115. Vyas D, Laput G, Vyas A. Chemotherapy-enhanced inflammation may lead to the failure of therapy and metastasis. Onco Targets Ther. 2014;(7):1015-1023.

116. Rusu RA, Sîrbu D, Curseu D, et al. Chemotherapy-related infectious complications in patients with hematologic malignancies. J Res Med Sci. 2018;23(68).

117. Wang X, Wei L, Xie X. Energy imbalance and cancer: Cause or consequence? IUBMB. 2017;69(10):776-784.

118. Anand P, Kunnumakara A, Sundaram C, et al. Cancer is a preventable disease that requires major lifestyle changes. Pharm Res. 2008;25(9):2097-2116.

119. Tonorezos E, Jones L. Energy balance and metabolism after cancer treatment. Semin Oncol. 2013;40(6):745-756.

120. Scott D, Milles M, Black A, et al. Multidimensional rehabilitation programmes for adult cancer survivors (Review). Published online 2015.

121. Myrhaug H, Mbalilaki J, Kersting Lie N-E, Hansen T, Nordvik J. The effects of multidisciplinary psychosocial interventions on adult cancer patients: a systematic review and meta-analysis. Disabil Rehabil. Published online 2018.

122. American Cancer Society. Cancer Treatment & Survivorship: Facts & Figures 2019-2021. Published online 2019.

123. Ellahham S. Exercise before, during, and after cancer therapy: Expert analysis. Published online 2019.

124. Nakano J, Hashizume K, Fukushima T, et al. Effects of aerobic and resistance exercises on physical symptoms in cancer patients: A meta-analysis. Integr Cancer Ther. 2018;17(4):1048-1058.

125. Campbell K, Winters-Stone K, Wiskemann J, et al. Exercise guidelines for cancer survivors: Consensus statement from international multidisciplinary roundtable. 2019;51(11):2375-2390.

126. Stout N, Brown J, Schwartz A, et al. An exercise oncology clinical pathway: Screening and referral for personalized interventions. Cancer. Published online 2020.

127. Burr J, Jones L, Shephard R. Physical activity for cancer patients: Clinical risk assessment for exercise clearance and prescription. Can Fam Physician. 2012;58(9):970-973.

128. De Backer I, Schep G, Hoogeveen A, Vreugdenhil G, Kester A, van Breda E. Exercise Testing and Training in a Cancer Rehabilitation program: the advantage of the steep ramp test. Arch Phys Med Rehabil. 2007;88.

129. Steins Bisschop C, Velthuis M, Wittingk H, et al. Cardiopulmonary exercise testing in cancer rehabilitation: A systematic Review. Sports Med. 2012;24(5):367-379.

130. Braam K, Van Dulmen- Den Broefer E, Veening M, et al. Application of the steep ramp test for aerobic fitness testing in children with cancer. Eur J Phys Rehabil Med. Published online 2014.

131. Mayo J, Kravitz L. Fitness assessment part 3: Muscle strength and endurance. Personal Trainer. 1997;8.

132. Schneider C, Hsieh C, Sprod L, Carter S, Hayward R. Cancer treatment-induced alterations in muscular fitness and quality of life: the role of exercise training. Ann Oncol. 2007;18(12):1957-1962.

133. Durnin J, Womersley J. Body fat assessed from total body density and its estimation from skinfold thickness: measurements on 481 men and women aged from 16 to 72 years. Br J Nutr. 1974;(32):77.

134. Norton K, Norton L, Sadgrove D. Position statement on physical activity and exercise intensity terminology. J Sci Med Sport. 2010;(13):496-502.

135. de Souza A, da Silva L, Fayh A. Nutritional intervention contributes to the improvement of symptoms related to quality of life in breast cancer patients undergoing neoadjuvant chemotherapy: A randomized clinical trial. Nutrients. 2021;13:589.

136. Özlem Gür E, Nuri Dilek O, özsay O, et al. Factors affecting the postoperative morbidity in patients who underwent gastric or colorectal resection due to cancer: Does preoperative nutritional status affect postoperative morbidity? Clin Sci Nutr. 2019;(1):1.

137. Verdeja-Robles C, Cisneros-Sandoval J. Nutritional intervention and quality of life in cancer patients. Open Access J Cancer Clin. 2019;1(101).

138. Hwa Jung G, Hye Kim J, Sung Chung M. Changes in weight, body composition, and physical activity among patients with breast cancer under adjuvant chemotherapy. Eur J Oncol Nurs. 2019;44.

139. de las Penas R, Majem M, Perez-Altozano J, et al. SEOM clinical guidelines on nutrition in cancer patients (2018). Clin Transl Oncol. 21:87-93.

140. Muscaritoli M, Arends J, Bachmann P, et al. ESPEN practical guideline: Clinical nutrition in cancer. Clin Nutr. Published online 2021:2898-2913.

141. Roza AM, Shizgal HM. The Harris Benedict equation reevaluated: resting energy requirements and the body cell mass. Am J Clin Nutr. 1984;40(1):168-182.

142. Gariballa S, Forster S. Energy expenditure of acutely ill hospitalised patients. Nutr J. 2006;5(9).

143. Massarini S, Ferrulli A, Ambrogi F, et al. Routine resting energy expenditure measurement increases effectiveness of dietary intervention in obesity. Acta Diabetol. 2018;55:75-85.

144. Barrera S, Demark-Wahnefried W. Nutrition during and after cancer therapy. Oncology. 2009;23(2):15-21.

145. Kushi L, Doyle C, McCullough M, et al. American cancer society guidelines on nutrition and physical activity for cancer prevention: Reducing the risk of cancer with healthy food choices and physical activity. Ca Cancer J Clin. 2012;62(1).

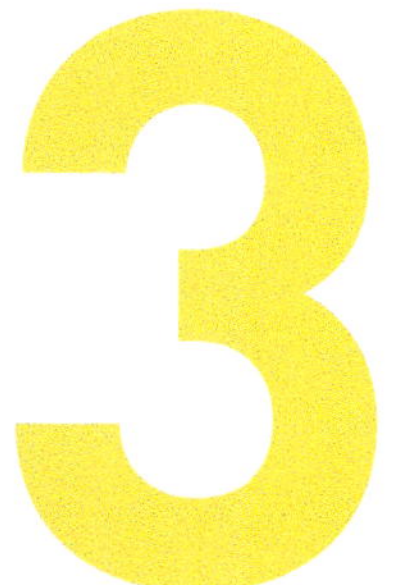

3 ANATOMY OF THE LYMPHATIC SYSTEM

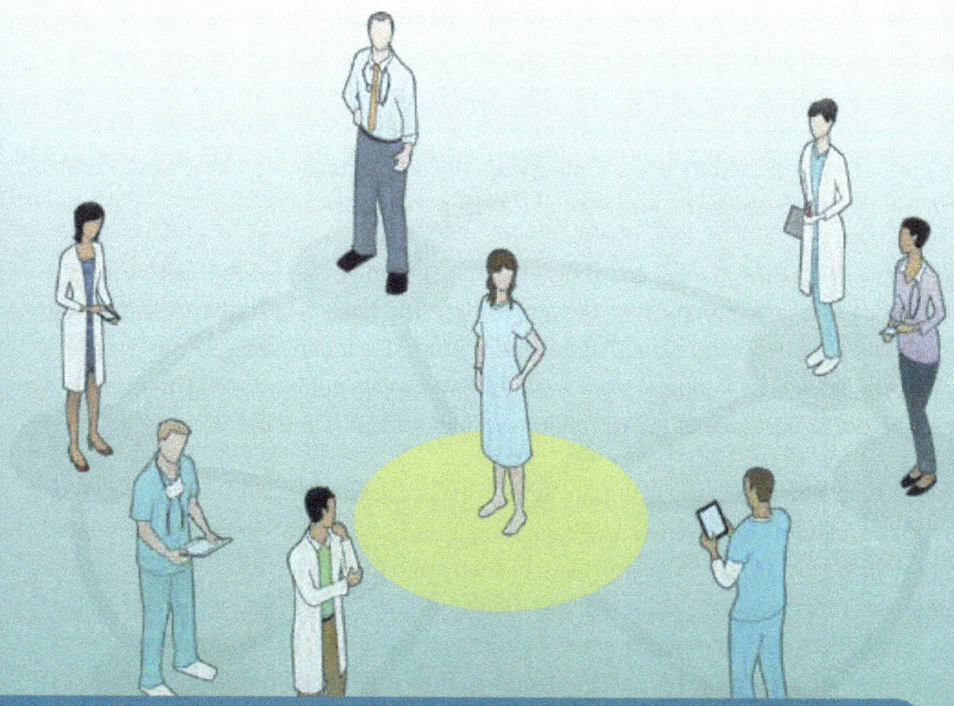

3.1   INTRODUCTION

The earliest references to the lymphatic system probably date back to the era of Hippocrates (460-370 BC) and Aristoteles (384-322 BC).[1] In these early references, sporadic observations of a colourless or white fluid in vein-like structures were done without any knowledge concerning function or physiology. In ancient references these structures are often referred to as the 'white veins'.[2] Despite several accidental discoveries, the anatomy and function of the lymphatic system were neglected for about 2,000 years.[3]

In the Middle Ages the lymphatic system was rediscovered. Bartholomeus Eustachius (1520-1574), amongst others, wrote about the 'vena alba thoracis' or the white vein of the thorax. This structure is known today as the **ductus thoracicus, or thoracic duct**. Additionally, Eustachius discovered the connection between the 'vena alba thoracis' and the left subclavian vein, yet he was clueless about its function. The next important discovery was done by Gasparo Aselli (1581-1626). He did extensive research on dogs. In one experiment in which he killed the dogs after they had had a final meal, he discovered a network of white veins coming from the dog's intestines, the lacteals. He was also the first to describe the presence of valves in the 'white veins'.[2,4]

Eventually, it was the Danish anatomist Thomas Bartholin (1616-1680) who used the terminology 'vasa lymphatica' in his publication. His fame and authority led to the worldwide adoption of the lymphatic nomenclature. Bartholin was also the 'first' (it's debatable since Olaf Rudbeck from Sweden had similar publications at the time) to describe the importance of the lymphatics in fluid transport and pathology.[2]

After the introduction of the lymphatic system by Bartholin, many discoveries regarding lymphatic anatomy emerged. In the beginning, these anatomical findings were related to specific bodily areas. An overall view of the lymphatic system was still lacking. The Hunter brothers (Wiliam 1718-1783 and John 1728-1793) investigated the mapping of the lymphatic system in many animals by using mercury injections. They also demonstrated the absorbing capacity of the lymphatics. It was Paolo Mascagni (1755-1815) who refined the technique of mercury injections and was able to describe the bigger part of the lymphatic system in his atlas *Vasorum lymphaticorum*.[2,4]

The following important discoveries are related to the spread of malignant cells by the lymphatic system. Rudolf Virchow (1821-1902) drew attention to the importance of the lymph nodes as they serve as a sort of filter and defense mechanism. He actually laid out the fundamentals of the sentinel procedure (which became common clinical practice in 2001).[2,4]

Despite all the discoveries related to the anatomy of the lymphatic system, it was not until 1896, when Ernest Starling (1866-1927) published his paper on fluid exchange across capillary membranes, that any insights into lymphatic physiology arose. Apart from the fluid exchange, Starling also contributed to the pathophysiological insights on edema formation. Roughly parallel with these physiological discoveries, the embryological development of the lymphatic system also came to light, with Florence Sabin (1871-1953) publishing *The origin and development of the lymphatic system* in 1913. She described the close relationship between the veins and lymphatics (a lot of similarities between veins and lymph vessels exist e.g., presence of valves, three-layered wall, ...). Early in embryological development, three pairs of lymphatic sacs are formed around day 36 (which is two weeks after the start of the cardiovascular system). Next, the lymphatic vessels are formed, first in close proximity to the large arteries, with the smaller vessels developing after that.[5]

Further major advancements with respect to the lymphatic system were achieved by the introduction of new imaging techniques like lymphography, lymphoscintigraphy and lymphofluoroscopy.[6-8] These techniques made it possible to do in vivo investigations of the lymphatic systems. Many of these techniques have led to the current knowledge on lymphatic functioning, lymphatic disease and lymphatic anatomy.

3.2 THE LYMPHATIC SYSTEM

3.2.1 General considerations

The anatomy of the lymphatic system will be discussed from that point of view that will allow you to understand the anatomy in relation to the treatment approaches that are discussed in the other chapters. It is by no means the intent to offer a complete overview, in detail, of the anatomy of the lymphatic system.

The lymphatic system is composed of the lymphatic organs, on the one hand, and the lymphatic vessels, on the other hand. The lymphatic organs, both primary and secondary, as described in table 3.1, play a very important role in the body's immune defense. Despite the importance of a properly working immune defense system, it will not be discussed any further here. Another important function of the lymphatic system is to enable the uptake of dietary lipids and proteins and other large chains molecules by the lacteals in the intestines; this will not be discussed in detail either. From a practical point of view, the focus on the anatomy of the lymphatic vessels will be on their transporting capacity. It is therefore important to understand how the different lymph vessels are distributed in the body and the important key features of the different vessel types. Additionally, it is also important to have knowledge of the interaction between the lymph vessels and the lymph nodes. The lymphatic vessels will be discussed from the smallest vessels to the largest vessels, according to the lymphatic flow that needs to be established. The lymph nodes of the most important areas, axilla – breast – head and neck – groin and pelvis, will be discussed in detail as well.

Primary lymphatic organs	Secondary lymphatic organs
• Bone marrow (→ B-lymphocytes) • Thymus (→ T-lymphocytes)	• Lymph nodes • Spleen • MALT (mucosa lymphatic tissue) • BALT (bronchus lymphatic tissue • GALT (gut lymphatic tissue) • Peyer's patches • Tonsils

Table 3.1   Primary and secondary lymphatic organs.

In general, both topographically and functionally, three distinct types of lymphatic systems can be found in the human body.

- Most superficial, the **epifascial systems** drains the interstitial fluid from the skin, subcutis and connective tissue.
- Underneath the fascia, the **deep or subfascial lymphatic system** can be found. The subfascial system drains the interstitial fluid from the muscles, joints and connective tissue. Collectors of the deep system often run along and within the neurovascular bundles. The epifascial and the subfascial system are interconnected by perforating vessels. Within each system, anastomoses occur between different vessels, enhancing collateral flow.
- Thirdly, the **organ collectors** and **lacteals** drain the interstitial fluid from the different organs and are involved in the uptake of large dietary molecules.

The lymphatic vessels start at the level of the interstitial space around the microcirculation. The lymphatic network begins with microscopic vessels called lymphatic capillaries or initial lymphatics in the tissues. Since the lymphatic vessels are not interconnected with the vascular capillaries, it is said that the lymphatics start in a blind manner. The smallest lymphatics are called lymph capillaries or initial lymphatics. These closed-ended tubes have a wall that consists of a single layer of endothelial cells. The lymph capillaries lack a basement membrane and have overlapping endothelial cells that are joined by loose junctions. Additionally, the endothelial cells are anchored to the surrounding tissue by collagen filaments called anchoring filaments. These anchoring filaments keep the capillaries in place and help the capillaries with the uptake of interstitial fluid. When the interstitial space fills with fluid the tension on the anchoring filaments increases and the loose junctions of the endothelial cells will open.

It is important to note that although the opening of the loose junctions can be seen as a valve function, the lumen of the lymphatic capillaries has no valves at all. Therefore, the lymph fluid can move freely within the lymphatic capillaries; at this level no unidirectional flow has yet been established.

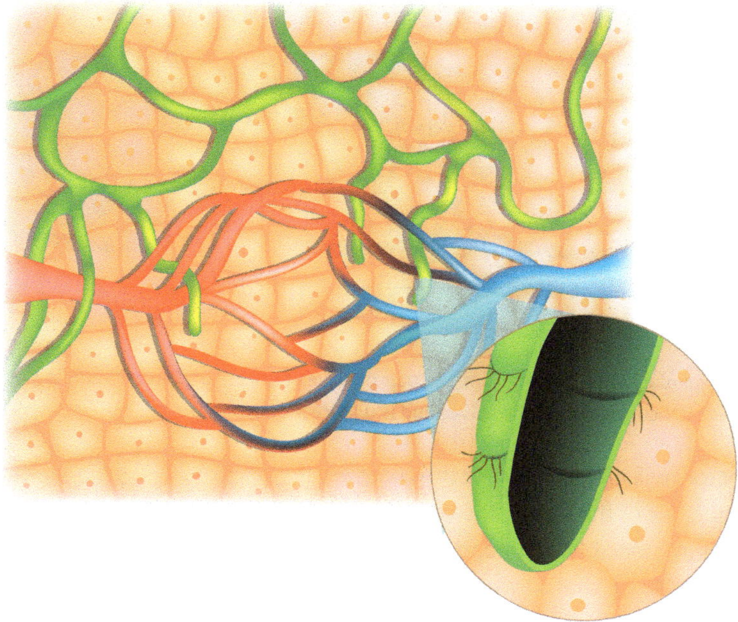

A schematic representation of the interaction between blood capillaries (microcirculation) and the initial lymphatic vessel. The connection between the blood capillaries and lymphatic capillaries is absent, hence a blind start of the lymphatic system. In the magnification, the loose junctions are clearly visible as well as the anchoring filaments that hold the lymphatic capillary in place and aid in the filling process of the lymphatic capillaries.

Lymphatic capillaries will merge to form larger lymphatic vessels. From the capillary bed onwards, the next type of lymphatic vessels are called pre-collectors. Gradually the pre-collectors, which are still small (approximately 15 μm in diameter), will evolve from a single layer of endothelium cells to a three-layered (three tunics) vessel wall. The tunica intima is the single layer of endothelial cells. The tunica intima has flaps, which are protrusions from the endothelial cells, that will act as valves. Due to the presence of these valves, a unidirectional flow is now established. The tunica media is a layer of smooth muscle cells covering the tunica intima. The smooth muscle cells are wrapped spirally around the intima, which makes them suitable for propelling lymph fluid in a peristaltic fashion. The smooth muscle has an autonomic contraction frequency. Additionally, this contraction frequency can increase based on a myogenic stretch reflex. This stretch reflex acts as a protection towards the overfilling (which can cause damage to the vessel) of the segments. The tunica adventitia is the third layer and consists of loose collagenous connective tissue and receives the innervation and blood supply of the vessels. With the presence of the valves, the lymph vessels can be divided into segments from one pair of valves to the next. Such a segment is called a lymphangion, which can be viewed as the functional unit of a lymph vessel.

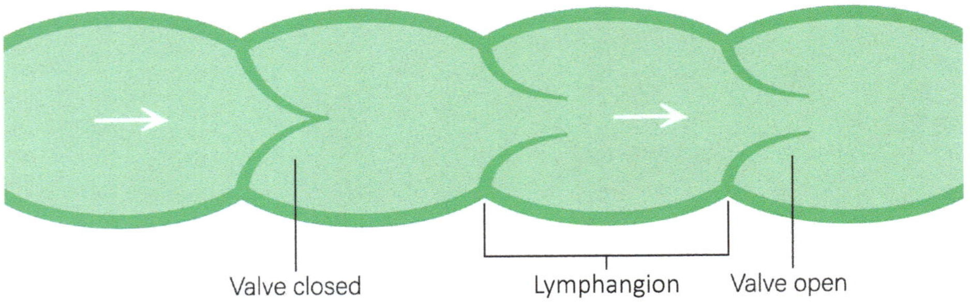

Figure 3.2 Presentation of a lymphangion, from one pair of valves to the next. Direction of flow is organized by the insertion of the valves and is unidirectional.

Next, the pre-collectors will interconnect to the collectors. While the pre-collectors run from the capillary bed out of the tissue, the collectors are larger lymph vessels running rectilinear towards a cluster of lymph nodes. The collectors have an increased lumen as well (between 100-600 µm) and a three-layered wall that is built alike the wall of the pre-collectors. However, the tunica media (smooth muscle) of the collectors is more pronounced in comparison to the pre-collectors, enhancing the transport capacity of the collector. Once a collector reaches a cluster of lymph nodes, it will interconnect with a chain of lymph nodes. As stated earlier, the transport of lymph fluid starts blindly at the interstitial space. Therefore, the fluid that is being transported by the lymph vessels from the interstitial space towards the clusters of lymph nodes can be contaminated with pathogens but may also contain death cells (like red blood cells) and end products of regeneration processes. It is of the utmost importance that the 'contaminated' lymph fluid does not enter the blood stream (due to the risk of a systemic infection/ outbreak). Therefore, the lymph nodes have the essential task of filtering the lymph fluid originating from the tissues. As mentioned, clusters of lymph nodes can be found in strategic places like the groin, pelvis, intestines, axilla and neck region of the human body (figure 3.3). A human body can have up to 1,500 lymph nodes.[9]

Afferent collectors bring the 'contaminated' fluid to the bean-like shaped lymph node (figure 3.4). The afferent collectors will enter the lymph node at the convex part of the bean shape and the efferent lymph vessel will leave the lymph node at its concavity. The concavity also receives the neurovascular bundle of the lymph node. Due to the composition of a lymph node as well as the discrepancy between the number of afferent collectors (many) and efferent collectors (few), lymph flow is decreased significantly.

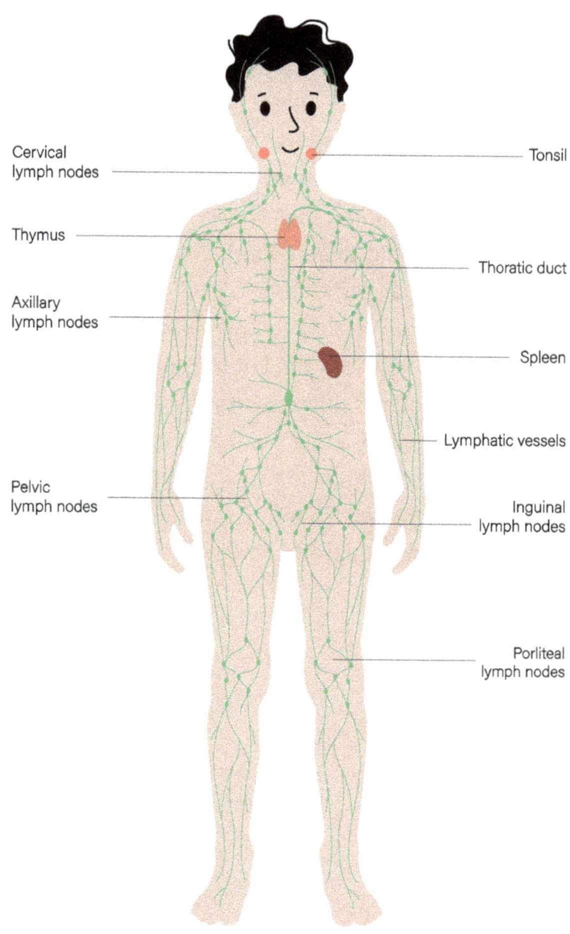

Figure 3.3   Schematic view of the body regions with strategic clusters of lymph nodes.

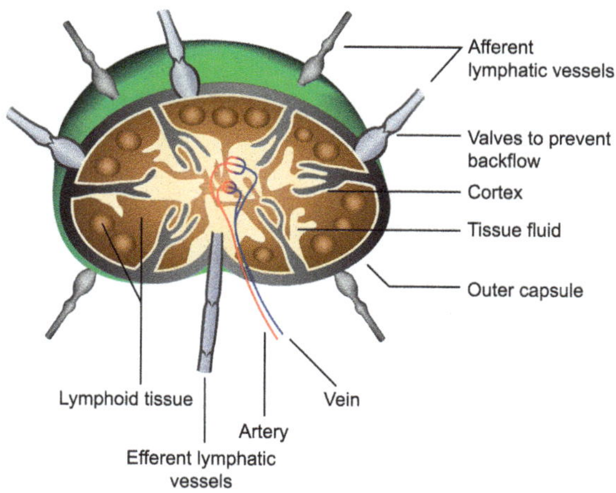

Figure 3.4   Schematic view of a single lymph node.

A lymph node is composed of trabeculae and medulla. The trabeculae act as a labyrinth, providing time for the medulla to filter the lymph fluid. Once the lymph fluid is filtered it is redirected towards the efferent collectors. These efferent collectors will merge into lymphatic trunks. Lymphatic trunks will transport the clean lymph fluid towards the confluence of the lymphatic system and the blood circulation. The biggest lymphatic trunk is called the thoracic duct. The thoracic duct (figure 3.5) is fed by the collectors from the lower half of the body (all fluid originating below the umbilicus) and starts between the level of the second lumbar vertebra and 9th thoracic vertebra. It ascends into the posterior mediastinum and runs (in most cases, 95%) towards the left venous angle created by the left subclavian vein and the left internal jugular vein. In 5% of the cases the endpoint of the thoracic duct is different, for instance both right and left venous angle or solely into the right venous angle. As the thoracic duct runs through the thorax, additional trunks interconnect with it. In this way, the thoracic duct also receives clean/filtered lymph fluid that originated from the upper left quadrant of the body and neck. A description of the lymphatic anatomy in detail can be found in Földi's *Textbook of lymphology*.[10]

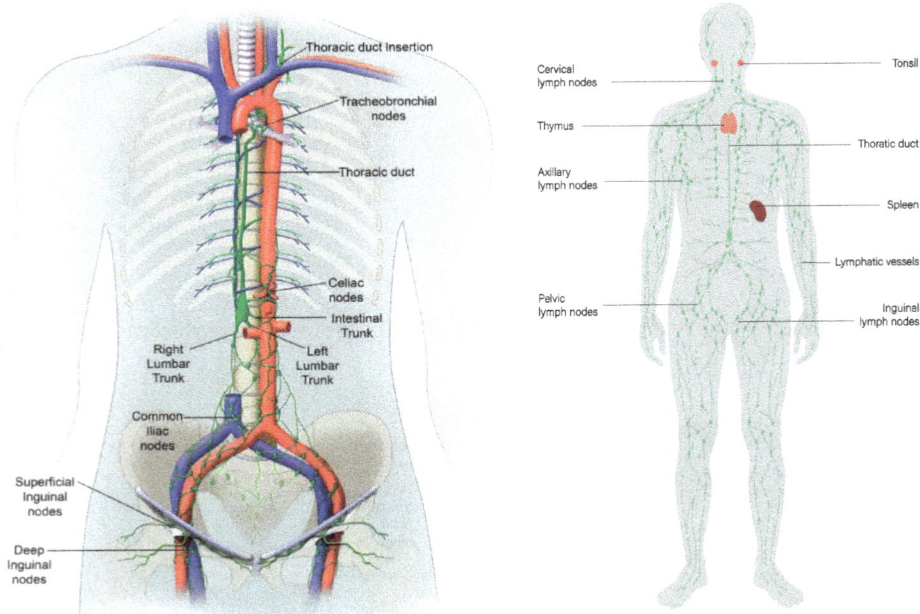

Figure 3.5 Schematic view of the course of the thoracic duct.

In figure 3.6, a schematic overview is provided concerning the return of lymph fluid to the blood circulation. About 75% of the lymph fluid is returned at the level of the left venous angle and 25% is returned by the right venous angle.

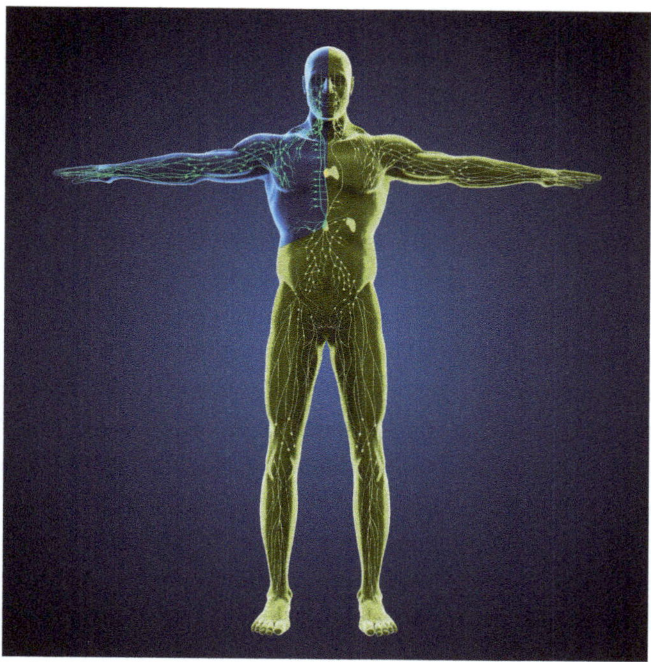

Figure 3.6   A schematic representation of the drainage of lymph fluid towards the circulatory system.

3.2.2   Important clusters of lymph nodes

Thus far, the anatomy has been discussed in a general way. Next, some essential details regarding the anatomy, especially the organization of the clusters of lymph nodes, will be discussed. These details will allow you to gain better insight into the possible formation of lymphedema after surgery (especially cancer treatment) or other therapies in these areas, like radiation therapy, that can damage the lymphatic system or hamper its regeneration. We will focus on two distinct regions, the shoulder-breast-neck area and groin-pelvic area, since these areas are most commonly involved in surgery with lymph node removal. Of course, lymph nodes in other parts of the body can be excised/radiated as well, but that goes beyond the scope of this textbook.

3.2.2.1   Clusters of the axilla-breast-neck area

At the level of the axilla, thorax/breast and neck different clusters of lymph nodes can be defined based on their topographical location.[11-13]

- The lateral or brachial cluster is situated on the inferior-medial side of the axillary vein. Its afferent collectors drain the lymph fluid from the superficial and deep compartments of the arm. Some superficial collectors of the arm run alongside the cephalic vein. The efferent collectors of the brachial cluster interconnect with the central or apical groups, while others pass into the supraclavicular nodes.

- **The anterior or pectoral cluster** is located behind the pectoralis major muscle and along the lower border of the pectoralis minor muscle. This cluster receives afferent collectors from the skin and muscles of the anterior and lateral walls of the trunk above the umbilicus. It also drains the lateral parts of the breast. The efferent collectors interconnect with the central and apical clusters.
- **The posterior or subscapular cluster** is arranged as a chain that follows the subscapular vessels in the groove that separates the teres major and subscapularis muscles. The afferent collectors of this cluster collect the lymph fluid from the muscles and skin of the back and from the scapular area downwards to the iliac crest. The efferent collectors of this cluster drain into the central and apical clusters.
- **The central cluster** is located centrally in the adipose tissue between the posterior and anterior cluster. The efferent collectors interconnect with the apical cluster.
- **The apical cluster** is located in the apex of the axilla with the majority of the lymph nodes on the inferomedial part of the proximal end of the axillary vein. This cluster receives afferent collectors from all the other axillary clusters. The efferent collectors interconnect with the subclavian trunk to progress into the right lymphatic duct. On the left side of the body the efferent collectors interconnect with the thoracic duct.

Other important clusters to keep in mind concerning the breast are the **parasternal or internal thoracic cluster** and the **intercostal cluster.** The parasternal cluster receives the lymph fluid from the breast and afferents from the deepest parts of the anterior thoracic and abdominal walls above the umbilicus. The lymph fluid is passed on to the large trunks (right lymphatic duct, thoracic duct) or directly to the subclavian veins. The intercostal cluster's afferent collectors come from the satellites of the posterior intercostal arteries and their efferent collectors drain into the thoracic duct on the left, or into the right lymphatic duct.

> **Important note:**
> Axillary clearance as executed during breast cancer surgery can have three different magnitudes, referred to as a level I, II or III. These levels are not entirely parallel/similar to the description of the clusters of the axilla. During a level I procedure the lymph nodes under the lower edge of the pectoralis minor muscle are removed. During a level II procedure the lymph nodes under the lower edge of the pectoralis minor muscle **and** underneath the pectoralis minor muscle are removed. During a level III procedure the lymph nodes under the lower edge of the pectoralis minor muscle **and** underneath the pectoralis minor muscle **and** above the pectoralis minor muscle are removed.[14] This relationship between the levels of axillary clearance and the clusters of the axilla is shown in figure 3.7.

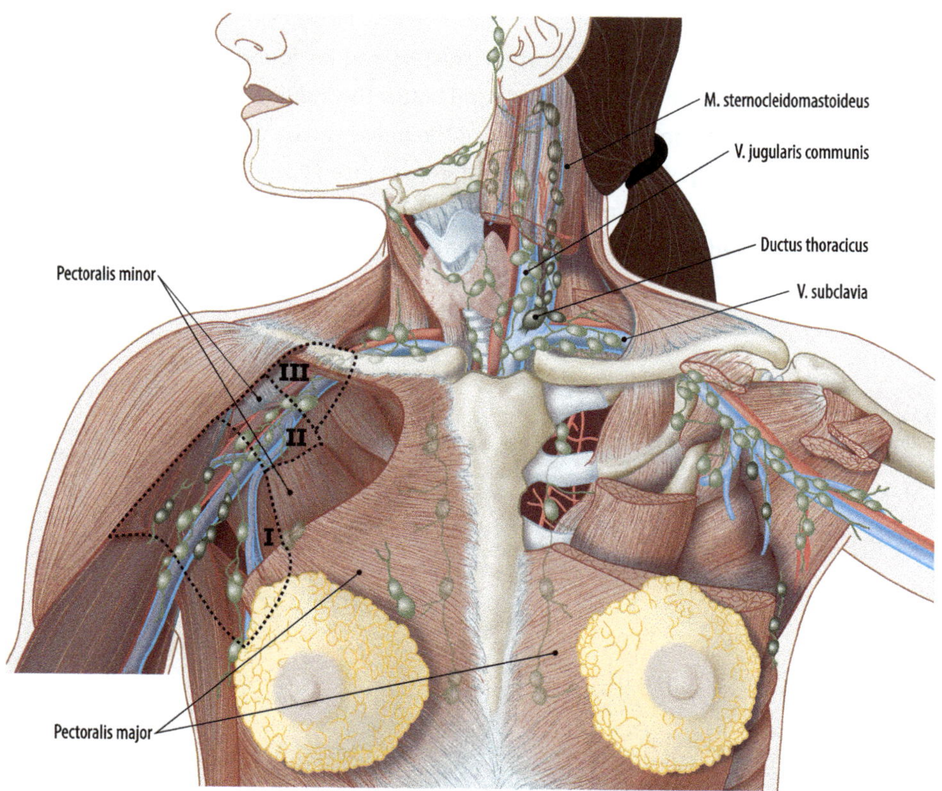

Figure 3.7 Lymphatic system of the axilla-breast-neck area.

In the pelvic and groin region, important clusters can be found both superficial and deep. Most of the superficial nodes are found below the inguinal ligament. Deep lymph nodes are found in the pelvis. The clusters of the pelvis can be divided into parietal and visceral clusters.[15,16] These areas are of great importance in understanding the damage that can be inflicted to the lymphatic system by surgery or radiation therapy. See figure 3.8 for a detailed overview of the different clusters.

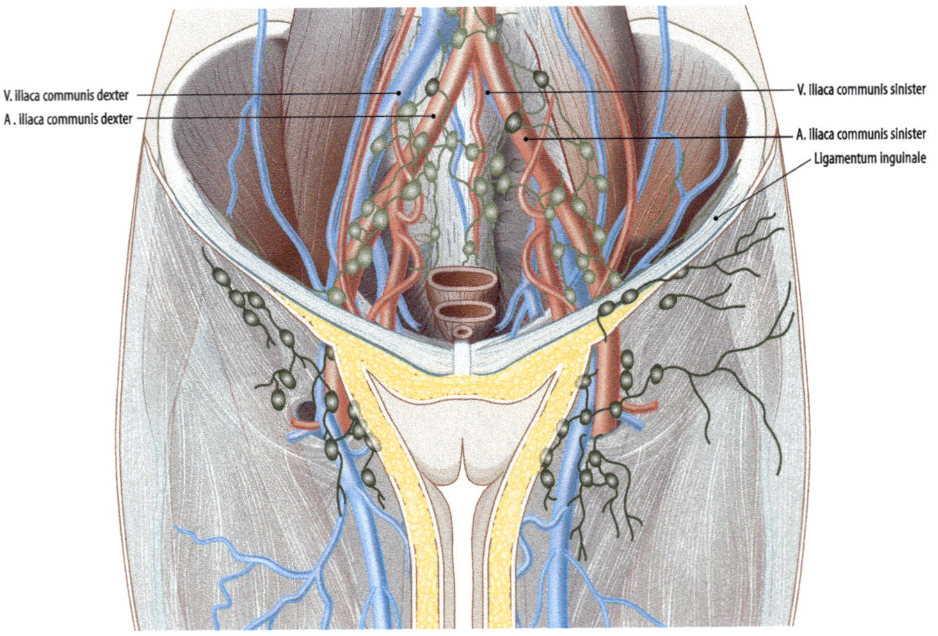

Figure 3.8   Lymphatic system of the groin and pelvic area.

Superficial clusters of the groin and pelvic area

The **superficial inguinal clusters** are one of the most important lymphatic clusters of the body. The lymph nodes are scattered in the space which is bounded superiorly by the inguinal ligament, laterally by the medial border of the sartorius muscle and medially by the upper border of the adductor longus muscle (area of the contributories of the great saphenous vein or Scarpa's triangle). By drawing a +sign on the terminus of the great saphenous vein, the superficial cluster can be divided into four subgroups. The horizontal line separates the cluster into the superior and inferior superficial inguinal lymph nodes. The vertical line subdivides the cluster into a medial and a lateral group of lymph nodes. The superficial clusters receive afferent collectors from the lower limb, pubic area, the area below the umbilicus (abdominal wall) and the lateral side of the thigh. The efferent collectors interconnect with the deep pelvic clusters by means of the saphenous opening or by perforating the cribiform fascia.

The **parietal clusters** are:
- the deep inferior epigastric cluster;
- the deep circumflex iliac cluster;
- the sacral cluster.

The parietal clusters drain lymph fluid from the anterior, lateral, posterior and inferior walls of the pelvis, the perineum and the muscles covering the pelvic girdle. Their efferent collectors interconnect with the external iliac clusters.

The **visceral clusters** are:
- The **juxtavisceral clusters** drain the lymph fluid from the bladder, in the urinary compartment of the pelvis, vagina, cervix, right and left aspects of the rectum, in the posterior digestive pelvic compartment. The efferent collectors interconnect with the external iliac, internal iliac or presacral clusters.
- The **external iliac clusters** can be divided into three chains: the lateral, intermediate and medial chain, respectively. These chains drain lymph fluid from the lower limb, penis/clitoris, obturator vessels, prostate gland, the fundus of the urinary bladder, the cervix uteri or the upper part of the vagina. The efferent collectors of each external iliac chain drain into the corresponding common iliac clusters.
- The **internal iliac clusters** drain the lymph fluid from the posterior part of the prostate gland, the lateral and lower parts of the urinary bladder, the membranous and prostatic segments of the urethra, the seminal vesicles, the middle and lower parts of the vagina, the body of the uterus and the middle part of the rectum. The efferent collectors interconnect with the intermediate group of common iliac clusters.
- The **common iliac clusters** can be divided into a lateral, intermediate and medial chain, respectively. The common iliac clusters receive the lymph fluid from the internal and external iliac clusters and interconnect with pre-aortic cluster.

With the background knowledge that the lymphatic system needs to secure the fluid transport from the interstitial space of the tissues and the knowledge that specific clusters of lymph nodes filter lymph fluid and safeguard immune responses, we can now focus on the drainage pathways of the lymph fluid.

A generalized view on lymphatic transport is that epifascial interstitial fluid will enter the superficial lymphatic system and will stay superficially until the first cluster of lymph nodes is reached. Likewise, subfascial interstitial fluid is drained by the deep lymphatic system and continues towards clusters of lymph nodes. After filtering, both superficial and deep systems will interconnect with the various trunks that are located deep and centrally. An overview of the lymphatic flow is provided on the following body charts (figure 3.9).[13,17-22]

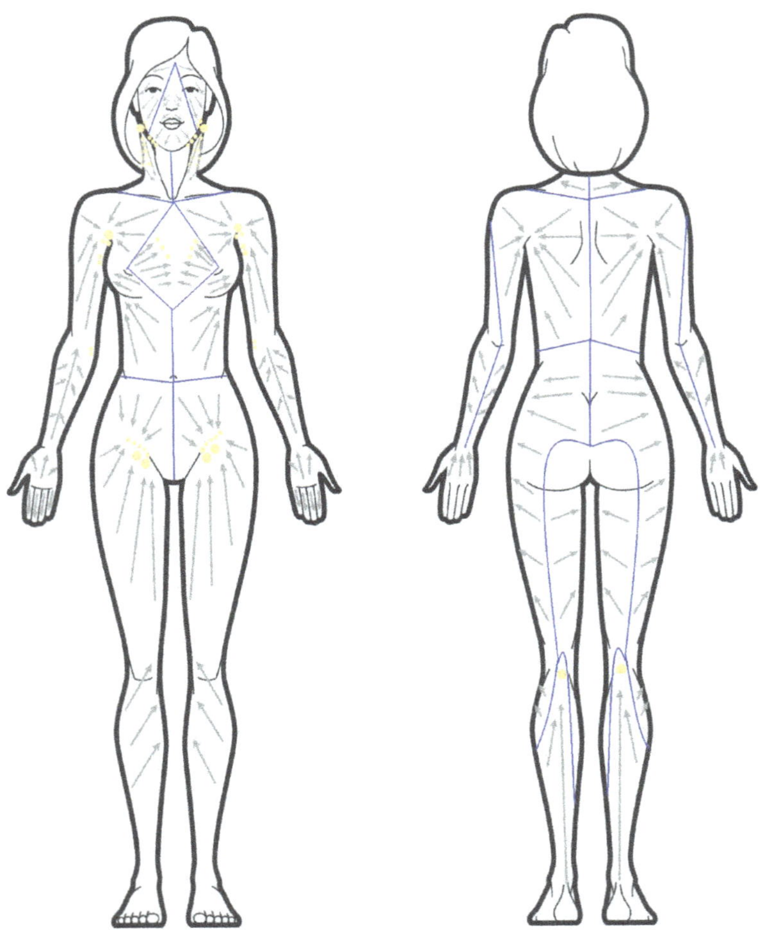

Figure 3.9 Simplified and schematic view of lymphatic transport based on scientific studies.

English terms	Nomina anatomica
Thoracic duct	Ductus thoracicus
Lymph node(s)	Nodus lymphaticus/ Nodi lymphatici
Subclavian vein	V. subclavia
Internal jugular vein	V. jugularis interna
Lumbar vertebra	Vertebra lumbalis
Thoracic vertebra	Vertebra thoracalis
Axillary vein	V. axillaris
Pectoralis major muscle	M. pectoralis major
Pectoralis minor muscle	M. pectoralis minor
Teres major muscle	M. teres major
Subscapularis muscle	M. subscapularis
Iliac crest	Crista iliaca
Posterior intercostal artery	A. intercostalis posterior
Inguinal ligament	Ligamentum inguinale
Sartorius muscle	M. sartorius
Adductor longus muscle	M. adductor longus
Great saphenous vein	V. saphena magna
Scarpa's triangle	Trigonum femorale mediale

3.3 REFERENCES

1. Crivellato E, Travan L, Ribatti D. The Hippocratic treatise 'On glands': the first document on lymphoid tissue and lymph nodes. Leukemia. 2007;21(4):591-592.
2. Lord RS. The white veins: conceptual difficulties in the history of the lymphatics. Med Hist. 1968;12(2):174-184.
3. Loukas M, Bellary SS, Kuklinski M, et al. The lymphatic system: a historical perspective. Clin Anat. 2011;24(7):807-816.
4. Irschick R, Siemon C, Brenner E. The history of anatomical research of lymphatics – From the ancient times to the end of the European Renaissance. Ann Anat. 2019;223:49-69.
5. Hong YK, Shin JW, Detmar M. Development of the lymphatic vascular system: a mystery unravels. Dev Dyn. 2004;231(3):462-473.
6. Abbaci M, Conversano A, De Leeuw F, Laplace-Builhé C, Mazouni C. Near-infrared fluorescence imaging for the prevention and management of breast cancer-related lymphedema: A systematic review. Eur J Surg Oncol. 2019;45(10):1778-1786.
7. Forte AJ, Boczar D, Huayllani MT, Lu X, Ciudad P. Lymphoscintigraphy for Evaluation of Lymphedema Treatment: A Systematic Review. Cureus. 2019;11(12):e6363.
8. Forte AJ, Boczar D, Huayllani MT, et al. Use of magnetic resonance imaging lymphangiography for preoperative planning in lymphedema surgery: A systematic review. Microsurgery. 2021.
9. Ackerman MJ. The Visible Human Project: a resource for anatomical visualization. Stud Health Technol Inform. 1998;52 Pt 2:1030-1032.
10. Földi EF, M. Földi's textbook of lymphology. 2012.
11. Lengelé B, Hamoir M, Scalliet P, Grégoire V. Anatomical bases for the radiological delineation of lymph node areas. Major collecting trunks, head and neck. Radiother Oncol. 2007;85(1):146-155.
12. Lengelé B, Nyssen-Behets C, Scalliet P. Anatomical bases for the radiological delineation of lymph node areas. Upper limbs, chest and abdomen. Radiother Oncol. 2007;84(3):335-347.
13. Suami H, Pan WR, Mann GB, Taylor GI. The lymphatic anatomy of the breast and its implications for sentinel lymph node biopsy: a human cadaver study. Ann Surg Oncol. 2008;15(3):863-871.
14. Krag DN, Anderson SJ, Julian TB, et al. Technical outcomes of sentinel-lymph-node resection and conventional axillary-lymph-node dissection in patients with clinically node-negative breast cancer: results from the NSABP B-32 randomised phase III trial. Lancet Oncol. 2007;8(10):881-888.
15. Gurdal SO, Kostanoglu A, Cavdar I, et al. Comparison of intermittent pneumatic compression with manual lymphatic drainage for treatment of breast cancer-related lymphedema. Lymphat Res Biol. 2012;10(3):129-135.
16. Lengelé B, Scalliet P. Anatomical bases for the radiological delineation of lymph node areas. Part III: Pelvis and lower limbs. Radiother Oncol. 2009;92(1):22-33.
17. Johnson AR, Granoff MD, Suami H, Lee BT, Singhal D. Real-Time Visualization of the Mascagni-Sappey Pathway Utilizing ICG Lymphography. Cancers (Basel). 2020;12(5).
18. Shinaoka A, Koshimune S, Suami H, et al. Lower-Limb Lymphatic Drainage Pathways and Lymph Nodes: A CT Lymphangiography Cadaver Study. Radiology. 2020;294(1):223-229.
19. Suami H. Lymphosome concept: Anatomical study of the lymphatic system. Journal of surgical oncology. 2017;115(1):13-17.
20. Suami H, Heydon-White A, Mackie H, Czerniec S, Koelmeyer L, Boyages J. A new indocyanine green fluorescence lymphography protocol for identification of the lymphatic drainage pathway for patients with breast cancer-related lymphoedema. BMC cancer. 2019;19(1):985.
21. Suami H, Koelmeyer L, Mackie H, Boyages J. Patterns of lymphatic drainage after axillary node dissection impact arm lymphoedema severity: A review of animal and clinical imaging studies. Surg Oncol. 2018;27(4):743-750.
22. Suami H, Scaglioni MF. Anatomy of the Lymphatic System and the Lymphosome Concept with Reference to Lymphedema. Semin Plast Surg. 2018;32(1):5-11.

4 PATHOPHYSIOLOGY OF CHRONIC EDEMA

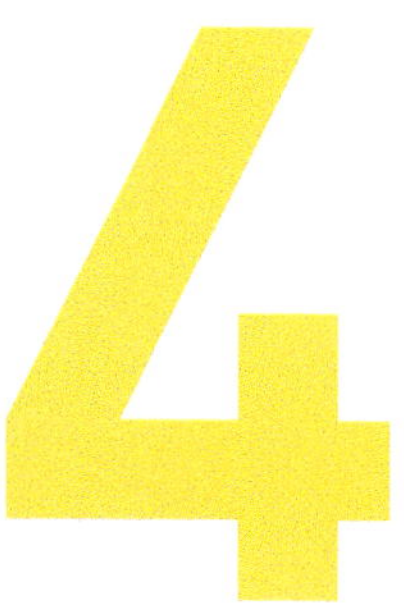

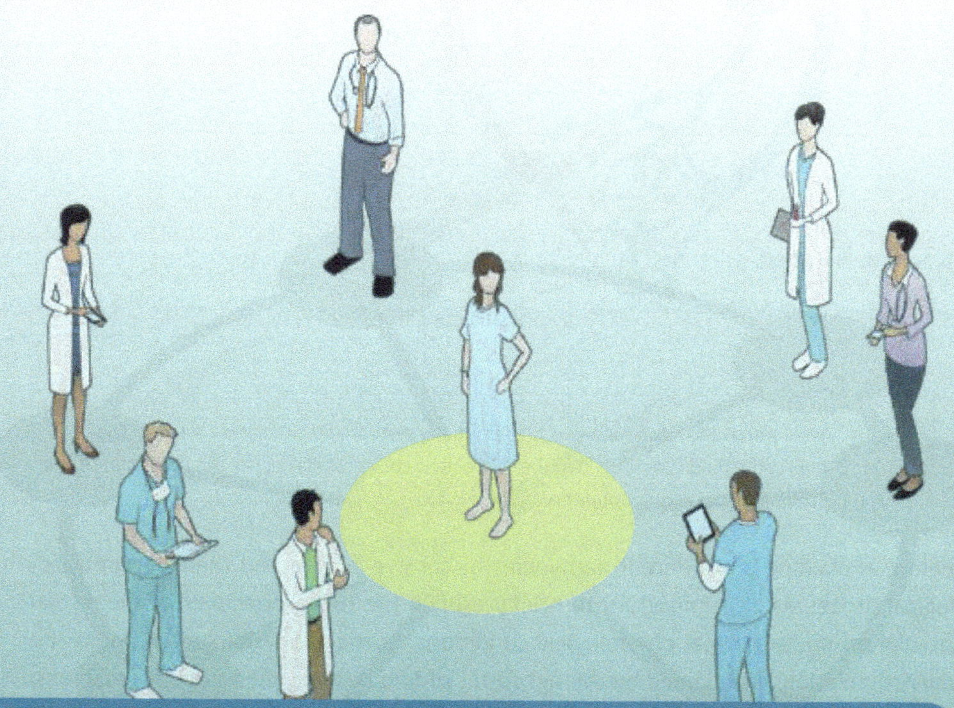

The learning objectives for this chapter are:

- Understanding the normal physiological processes of the microcirculation regarding fluid shifts
- Providing insight into the pathophysiological processes that can provoke swelling or chronic edema
- Providing insight into the different stages of chronic edema

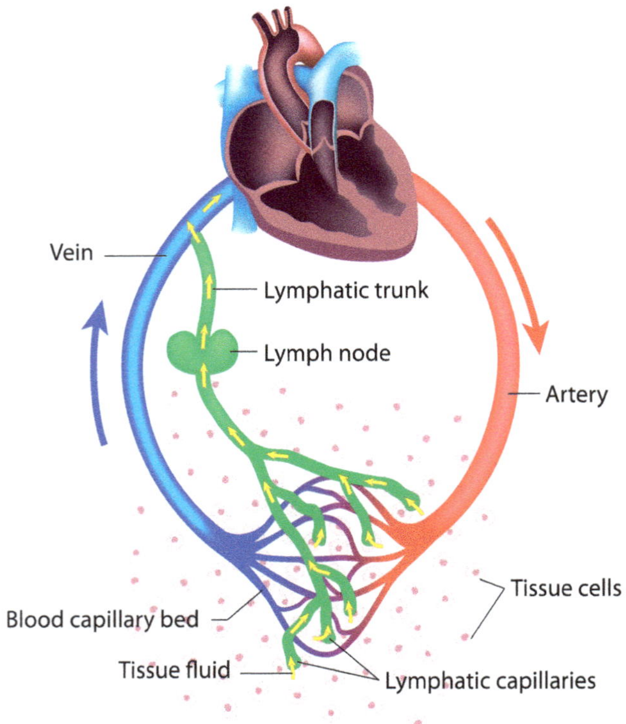

Figure 4.1 The interrelationship between the lymphatic system and circulatory system. The interstitial fluid is produced in the microcirculation (capillaries) as the net result of the Starling forces acting upon the capillary wall.

Before explaining the different aetiologies of chronic edema and their pathophysiological processes, it is important to briefly explain the ruling principles of the microcirculation under normal physiological conditions. In many physiology textbooks the microcirculation is explained by the net result of two distinct physiological processes, **filtration** and **(re)absorption,** respectively.[1] Filtration can be defined as the extravasation of plasma fluid through the capillary membrane and (re)absorption is the uptake of fluid from the interstitial area into the capillary. Although disclaimed for many years, this hypothesis of filtration and reabsorption is much too generalized and incorrect for many types of tissues, like subcutis, connective tissue, muscles, although these tissues account for up to 70% of human body mass. In some highly specialized tissues, absorption from the interstitial area is possible (e.g., intestines, kidneys). The relationship between filtration and reabsorption in tissues with respect to the different types of capillaries is shown in table 4.1 and figure 4.2. In most tissues continuous capillaries are found in the microcirculation. In specialized tissues the fenestrated and porous capillaries are found.

Continuous	Fenestrated	Porous
Small cell openings	Large cell openings	Large pores (30-40 µm)
Only diffusion of small molecules	Continuous basal membrane	RBC
Trancystosis for large molecules	Facilitation fluid fluxes	WBC
Most common type of capillary	Kidneys	Proteins
Muscle	Intestines	Spleen
Skin		Bone marrow
Subcutis and connective tissue		Liver

Table 4.1   Main characteristics of the different types of capillaries.

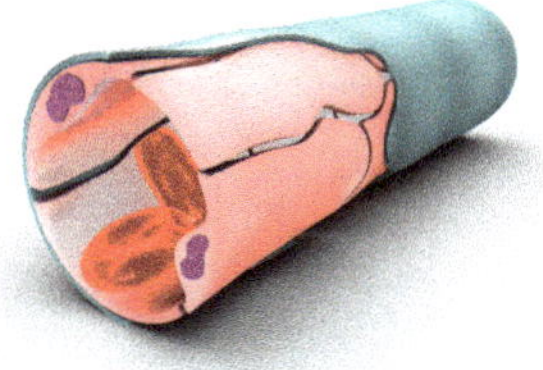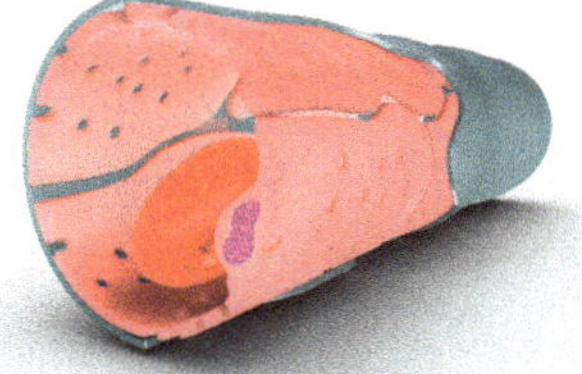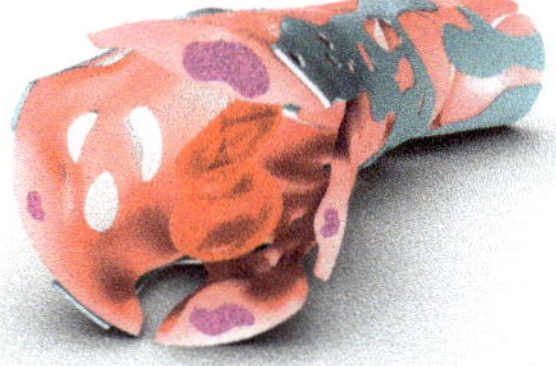

Figure 4.2   Different types of capillaries found in the human body. Left: continuous capillary. Middle: fenestrated capillary. Right: porous capillary.

Therefore, in tissues like the skin, the subcutis and muscle, there is only a net filtration of plasma exudate from the capillary towards the interstitial area. In normal microcirculation physiology it has been demonstrated that about 5-10% of the circulating plasma volume/24h escapes towards the interstitial space. Since there is a production of fluid within the interstitial space, the net result of the microcirculation is a filtration (fluid shift) towards the interstitial space. The net filtration is mainly influenced by four Starling forces:

- oncotic pressure within the capillary (πc);
- hydrostatic pressure within the capillary (Pc);
- oncotic pressure underneath the glycocalyx (πg);
- the tissue pressure, also assessed underneath the glycocalyx (Pg).

The actions performed by the starling forces on a capillary are depicted in figure 4.3.

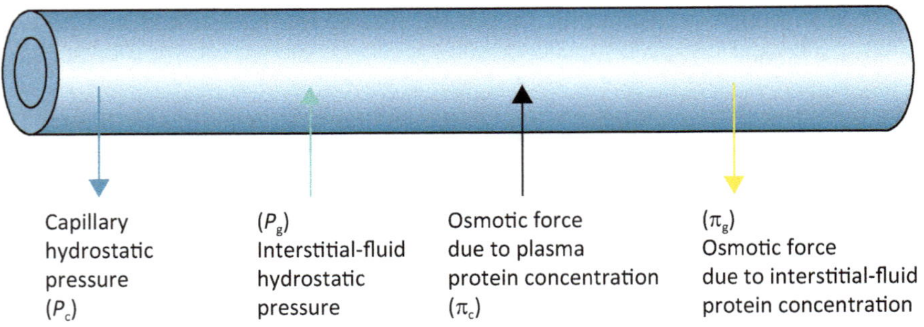

Capillary hydrostatic pressure (P_c)	(P_g) Interstitial-fluid hydrostatic pressure	Osmotic force due to plasma protein concentration (π_c)	(π_g) Osmotic force due to interstitial-fluid protein concentration

Figure 4.3 The Starling forces acting upon a capillary wall. The outward arrows denote the Starling forces that favor filtration and the inward arrows denote the Starling forces that favor reabsorption.

Therefore, the net filtration rate can be calculated using the **second revision (based on the discovery of glycocalyx)** of the Starling formula:[2]

$$Nf = Lp.S. \{(Pc - Pg) - \sigma(\pi c - \pi g)\}$$

In which:
- Nf = net filtration
- Lp = permeability of the capillary wall to water
- S = surface area available for filtration
- Pc = hydrostatic pressure (resulting from the blood pressure)
- Pg = tissue pressure assessed underneath the glycocalyx at the interendothelial cleft
- σ = Staverman's coefficient reflecting the permeability of the capillary wall for proteins
- πc = oncotic pressure within the capillary (mainly organized by the concentration of proteins, especially albumin)
- πg = oncotic pressure assessed underneath the glycocalyx at the interendothelial cleft

Note:
The glycocalyx is the inner liner of the endothelial cells in a blood vessel. The glycocalyx plays an important role in defining the permeability of a capillary (among others). The combination of the endothelial cells with the glycocalyx is called 'the endothelial surface layer'. Due to the discovery of the glycocalyx, the concentration of proteins is no longer assessed in the interstitial area; instead, it is measured within the interendothelial cleft. Hence, the second revision of the Starling formula.

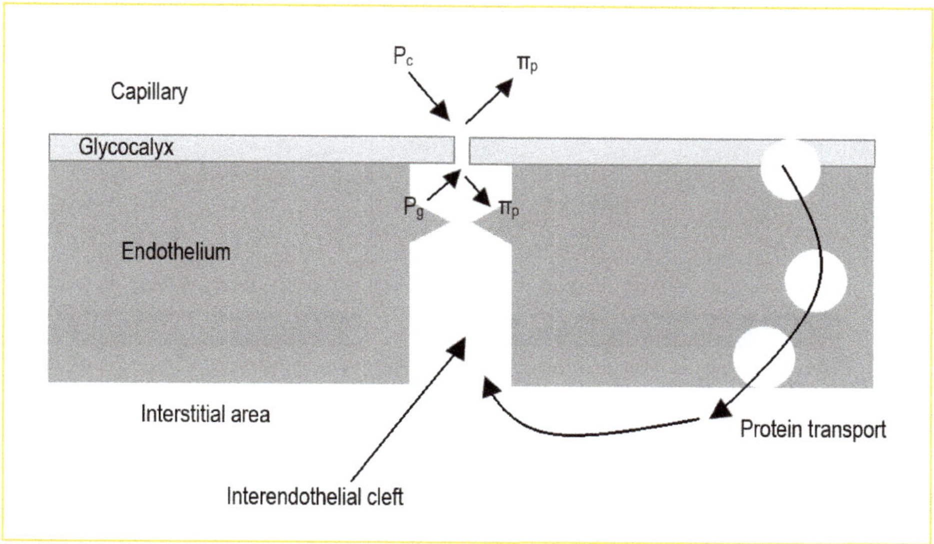

Figure 4.4 The impact of the glycocalyx on the assessment of the Starling Forces.

The net filtration formula is very important to understanding the pathophysiological changes that result in (chronic) edema. For instance, if π_c drops significantly (e.g., protein losing enteropathy), Nf will increase significantly, resulting in a steep rise of the lymphatic load. Once the lymphatic load exceeds the transport capacity of the lymphatic system, edema will arise.

Lymph production estimation for 24h
*4.7l x 1440 min (24h) = 6768l or between 3.35 – 6.7l of lymph (based on 5-10%)
*5.2l x 1440 min = 7488l or between 3.7 – 7.5l of lymph
→ Taking into account that 60% of the blood volume is plasma, a more detailed estimation of lymph production will be:
*4l (4.7l of blood is 2.82l of plasma) per 24h
*4.5l (5.2l of blood is 3.12l of plasma) per 24h

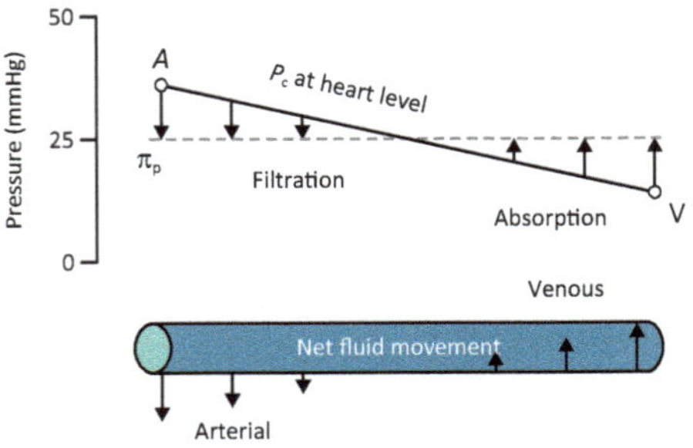

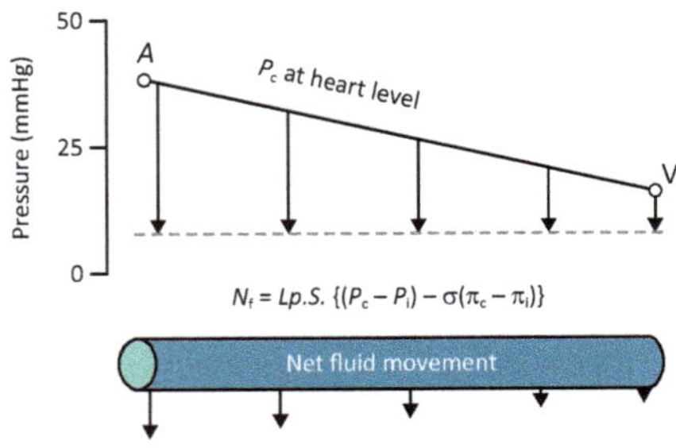

Starling hypothesized that if fluid would escape from the capillaries, an equilibrium needs to be established. Therefore filtration and absorption from the microcirculation should be equal.

Step 3: Second revision of the Starling with based upon the discovery of the glycocalyx

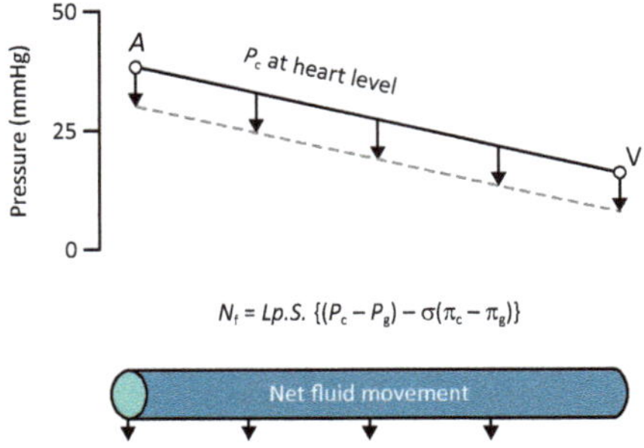

Figure 4.5 The different revisions of Starling's hypothesis (step 1) are depicted in three steps. In a first revision (step 2) net filtration was calculated by assessing the Starling forces in the capillary and in the interstitial area. Due to the discovery of the glycocalyx a second revision of the formula was made (step 3). In the second revision the Starling forces are assessed in the capillary and underneath the glycocalyx in the interendothelial cleft. Notice the changes in the second revision where i (interstiaital area) is replaced by g (glycocalyx).

Based on the aforementioned physiological principles, **chronic edema** can be seen as the accumulation of fluid (mostly water and a limited amount of proteins) within the interstitial space. Today, it is more common to talk about chronic edema instead of lymphedema. This change in definition has also led to a new taxonomy or classification of the different types of edema. We will therefore use the classification based upon pre-loading and after-loading edemas throughout the text. Chronic refers an edema that is present for more than six months and gets worse over time (e.g., increased swelling, additional skin changes).

Although this chapter focuses on edema formation, chronic edema is never a diagnosis, only a symptomatic presentation of an underlying cause of the edema. It is therefore very important to understand the different aetiologies that can have a chronic edema as a symptom. If these aetiologies can be treated, this should be attempted first. Chronic edema should only be treated if no other options for treatment are available, hence the importance of a multidisciplinary approach. First, rule out any treatable conditions; next, guide the patient toward the most appropriate treatment.

Remark:
Other classifications often found in the scientific literature are:
- pitting vs non-pitting edema;
- primary vs secondary lymphedema.

Remark:
The difference between swelling and edema is the duration in time. Chronic edema is present for at least six months and worsens over (although daily fluctuations in severity occur) time while a swelling is transient in nature. Swelling will resolve over time (from one day to several weeks).

4.2 PRE-LOADING CHRONIC EDEMA

A **pre-loading edema** can be defined as a chronic swelling due to an increased amount of interstitial fluid production and a normal transporting capacity of the lymphatic system. This normal lymphatic capacity is inadequate for absorbing and transporting all of the excess interstitial fluid. This pathophysiological condition occurs when there is an excessive hydrostatic pressure (e.g., varicose veins, PTS), and/or increased permeability (inflammation), and/or increased fragility (chronic venous insufficiency) within the microcirculation. Taking into account the second revision of the Starling formula, especially P_c, L_p are significantly increased. In case of hypoproteinemia (e.g., protein loosing enteropathy or hunger edema [Kwashiorchor]), π_c is significantly decreased. P_g can also be significantly decreased (e.g., myxedema), allowing much more filtration towards the interstitial space.

Examples of conditions that provoke pre-loading edema are:
- deep vein thrombosis (DVT);
- varicose veins (primary as well as secondary);
- post-thrombotic syndrome (PTS);
- chronic venous insufficiency (CVI);
- heart failure (right);
- myxedema (hypothyroidy, Graves disease, Hashimoto's thyroiditis);
- kidney failure.

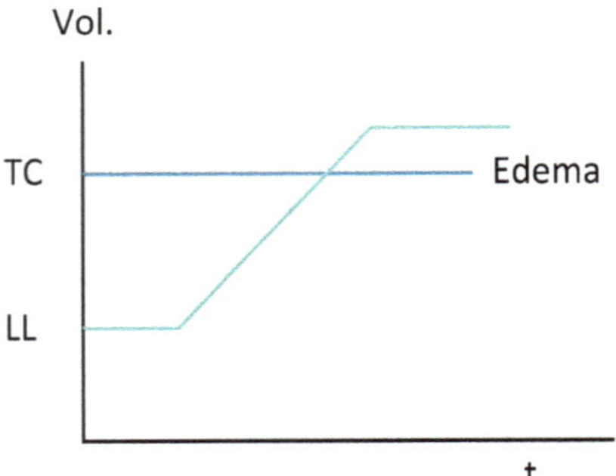

TC = Transport capacity
LL = Lymphatic load

Figure 4.6 Schematic explanation of the pathophysiology of a pre-loading edema.

4.3 AFTER-LOADING CHRONIC EDEMA

An **after-loading edema** can be defined as a chronic edema resulting from lymphatic incompetence. An after-loading edema is thus characterized by normal interstitial fluid production in combination with a decreased transport capacity of the lymphatic system. At the beginning of the condition, a normal physiological net filtration is apparent. Next, when interstitial fluid starts to accumulate, Pg will increase, creating a physiological constraint on the net filtration rate (self-limiting mechanism). This is the reason why an after-loading edema sets in slowly over time.

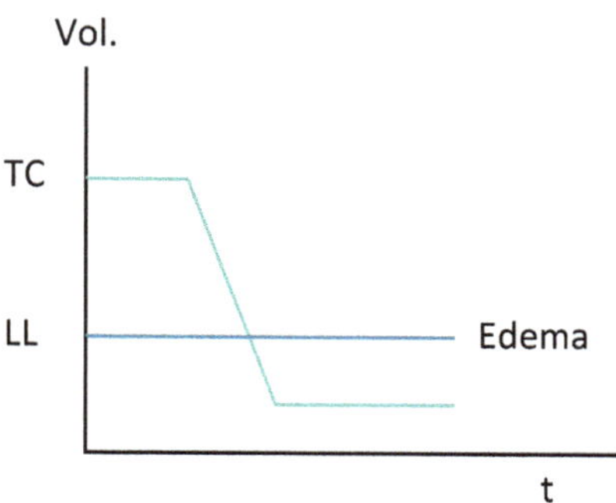

TC = Transport capacity
LL = Lymphatic load

Figure 4.7   A schematic explanation of an after-loading edema.

4.3.1 Primary and secondary lympathic disorders

The lymphatic disorders that are responsible for the after-loading edema can be of primary or secondary origin.

4.3.1.1 Primary lymphatic disorders

Primary disorders are innate or hereditary disorders that have a direct effect on the lymphatic system and its functionality (for examples of the primary causes of after-loading, see figure 4.8).

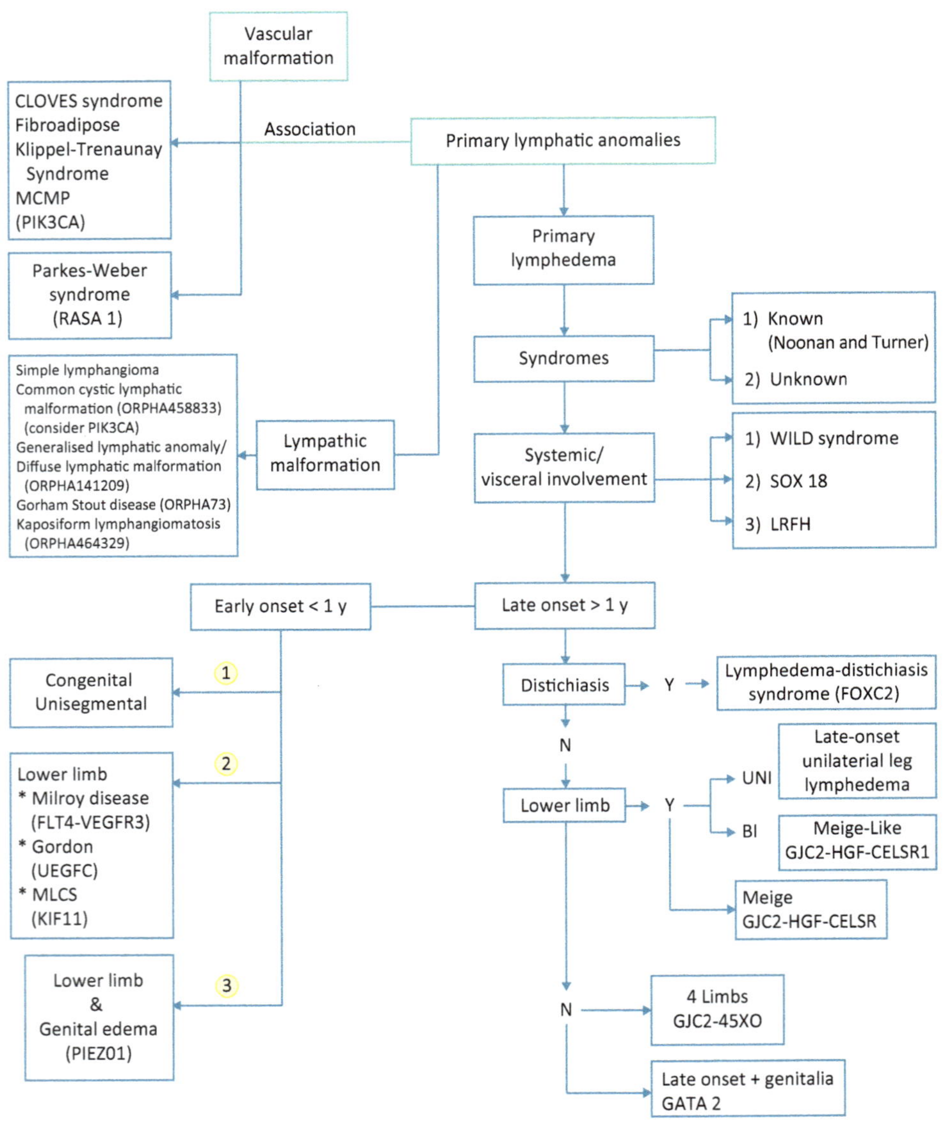

Based on Mortimer & Rockson, 2014, Clin J Invest.

Figure 4.8 Known causes of primary lymphedema and its genetic reason.

Primary causes of after-loading edema are rare (1/100,000) and are mostly seen in women. It can be present at birth or early after birth (within months to one year) or arise with a delay of many years. Primary lymphedema is thus divided into early-stage and late-stage onset, with the cut-off at 35 years of age.

Secondary lymphatic disorders (1/1000) that cause after-loading edema are provoked disorders due to surgery and other types of treatment, trauma, infections, cancer, etc. A well-known aetiology of a secondary lymphatic disorder is the cancer treatment-related lymphedema. Although cancer treatment-related lymphedema is the best-known cause and, in addition, the most investigated type of chronic edema, one should be aware that other aetiologies have a much higher incidence and are responsible for the largest number or patients suffering from chronic edema. An estimated 120 million people in tropical and subtropical areas suffer from lymphatic filariasis, representing a global prevalence of 2%. This type of secondary lymphedema is provoked by the parasite *Wuchereria bancrofti* (further explained in the section parasites). Additionally, the global LIMPRINT study has provided information and data about the different causes of chronic edema (see the results in table 4.3). This global study reveals that venous disease (pre-loading condition) and obesity are responsible for more cases of chronic edema than cancer-related chronic edema. With respect to cancer treatment-related chronic edema, an overview of the incidence/cancer diagnosis is provided in table 4.2.

Group	No. of studies	No. of patients	Pooled incidence %	Range	Random effects incidence %	95% CI
Overall	47	7779	15	0-73	15.5	11.0-21.0
Upper extremity	8	2130	3	1-39	5.1	1.1-17.9
Lower extremity	43	5456	20	1-66	19.9	14.3-26.8
Head and neck	3	139	4	0-8	NA	--
Melanoma (overall)	15	3676	9	1-66	16.3	8.6-27.8
• Upper	8	2130	3	1-39	5.1	1.1-17.9
• Lower	13	1546	18	6-66	28.0	17.2-42.2
Genitourinary (overall)	8	1060	11	1-23	10.1	3.2-25.2
• Bladder	2	267	16	15-23	16.2	0-100
• Penile	2	244	21	20-21	19.6	0-100
• Prostate	4	549	4	1-18	4.8	0.1-71.7
Gynecologic (overall)	22	2850	25	0-73	19.6	11.1-31.0
• Cervical	11	1544	27	2-49	21.8	11.6-35.8
• Endometrial	1	168	1	-	NA	--
• Vulvar	8	890	30	0-73	24.9	3.5-59-7
Sarcoma	1	54	30	-	NA	--

Table 4.2   Overview of the pooled incidence of cancer treatment-related lymphedema.

Condition	%
Venous disease	72.06
Obesity	54.41
Non-cancer other	14.71
Cancer	8.82
Treatment-related obstruction	8.82
Metastatic disease	8.82

Table 4.3 LIMPRINT study data. Causes of secondary chronic edema.[3-6]

Note:

It is important to understand that secondary lymphedema due to cancer treatment is the best studied cause of lymphedema. However, the patients that you will see in clinical practice are most commonly patients with venous disease, obesity and non-cancer related causes. Patients often have a mixed pathology, resulting in complex lymphatic cases.

4.3.2 Surgery and/or radiation therapy

A common and well-known cause of secondary lymphedema is surgery, whether or not combined with radiation therapy. During surgery, lymphatic vessels and especially lymph nodes can be resected or destructed, especially when the surgery is performed in areas at high risk for damage to the lymphatic systems. These areas at risk (see also Chapter 3) are the axilla, groin and pelvis, and the risk increases when surgery is performed in combination with a resection of lymph nodes.

In the case of cancer treatment, surgery is often followed by adjuvant therapies like radiation therapy or chemotherapy. Radiation therapy will destroy the newly formed lymphatics, which spectacularly increases the risk of edema formation.

4.3.3 Inflammation

Different types of infections can lead to damaged lymphatics. Benign lymphangitis can occur after insect bites or trauma. Normally, this inflammation has a natural course and will heal without any therapy. Malign lymphangitis occurs when bacteria are responsible for the inflammation. Treatment is based on the use of antibiotics.

A specific and severe bacterial induced infection is known as **erysipelas**. Erysipelas can cause the onset of chronic edema. Additionally, many patients suffering from chronic edema will experience an erysipelas infection due to skin breaks provoked by the edema. Erysipelas is the most feared type of infection. It is an infection provoked by streptococci or staphylococci. These bacteria can enter the body after skin breaks have appeared. These bacteria then become a systemic infection with rashes, high fever and nausea. Erysipelas is treated by antibiotics. If the erysipelas is recurrent, treatment becomes more difficult since bacteria will become resistant to the antibiotics. The infection itself can destruct parts of the lymphatic system. It is also known that patients with edema have a higher risk for an episode of erysipelas. Additionally, a first episode of erysipelas can cause chronic edema later on.[7]

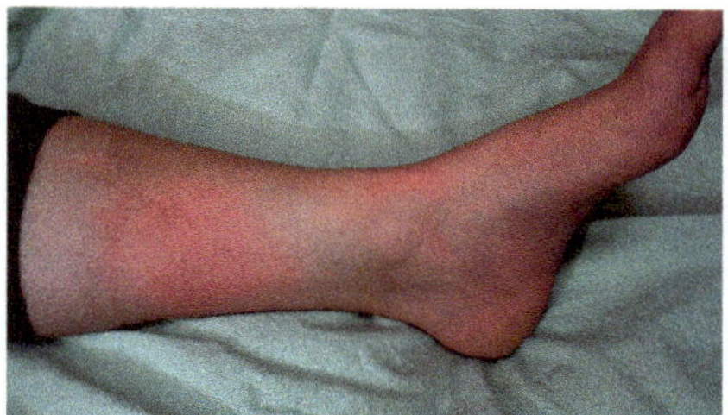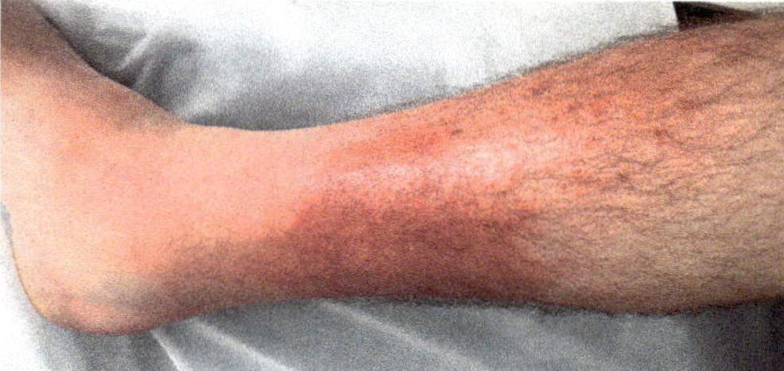

Figure 4.9   Examples of an Erysipelas infection.

4.3.4   Parasites

One might suspect that pre-loading edema or secondary lymphedema after cancer treatment are the most common aetiologies of chronic edema. Although true for Western countries, this is not the case worldwide. Worldwide, a parasite known as *Wuchereria bancrofti* is responsible for the highest number of patients with chronic edema, over 120 million patients. *Wuchereria bancrofti* is a parasite from the roundworm family. It is present in most tropical areas. The parasite enters the host (humans) via mosquito bites as well as through bathing in shallow and stagnant water. The microfilariae nest in the lymphatic system. Once they are full-grown, they block the collectors and impair lymphatic transport, causing chronic edema. In its adult stage, the parasite will produce microfilariae. These microfilariae spread into the blood stream. When a mosquito pricks a host, the microfilariae will enter its proboscis. When the mosquito takes its next blood meal from another host, the microfilariae leave the proboscis and enter the new host, provoking the next filariasis with concomitant edema.

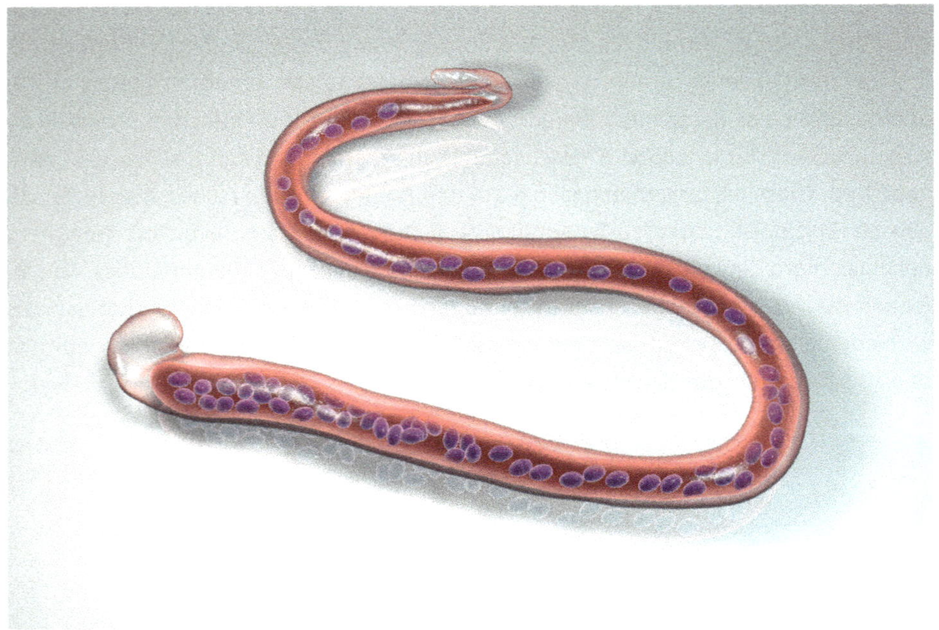

Figure 4.10 Example of the *Wurcheria bancrofti* parasite that causes filariasis lymphedema.

4.3.5   Neoplasms

It is not only the treatment of neoplasms that can cause swelling; neoplasms themselves can be responsible for swelling, as neoplasms grow within the lymphatic system or tumour growth blocks essential lymphatic pathways. Therefore, it is essential that an oncological work-up is performed upon suspicion of cancer.

Note:
Both pre-loading and after-loading edemas were discussed separately in this chapter. Bear in mind that many patients will have a chronic edema that is caused by multiple aetiologies, often with both pre-loading and after-loading causes.

4.4   STAGES OF CHRONIC EDEMA

Based upon the ISL2020 consensus document, chronic edema can be categorized into **four stages**:[8]

- stage 0 or subclinical edema;
- stage I;
- stage II;
- stage III.

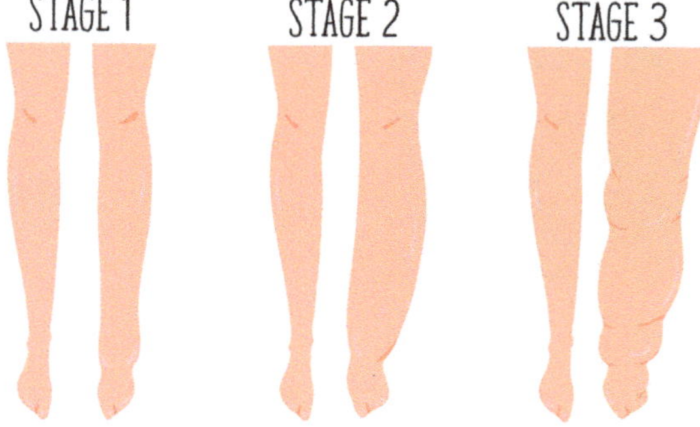

Figure 4.11   The final three stages of lymphedema.

4.4.1   Stage 0 or subclinical edema

Stage 0 can be defined as edema with deformations of the lymphatics, but no apparent (visible) swelling.

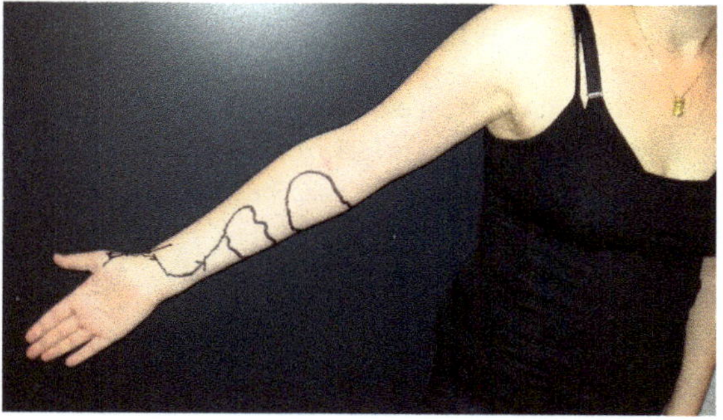

Figure 4.12   A patient with subjective feelings of lymphedema. The lymphatic damage was visualized by lymphofluoroscopy; circles are areas with 'splash' dermal backflow patterns. The lymphatic damage is limited and there is no visible swelling.

4.4.2   Stage I

A stage I edema is characterized by:

- an early accumulation of fluid relatively high in protein content (e.g., in comparison with 'venous' edema) which subsides with limb elevation;
- pitting may occur;
- an increase in various proliferating cells may also be seen.

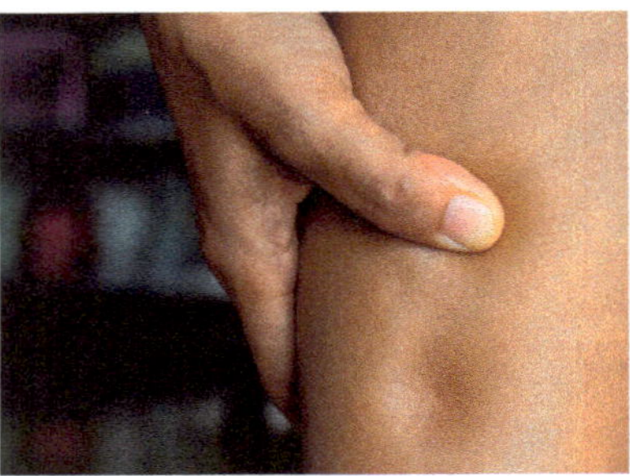
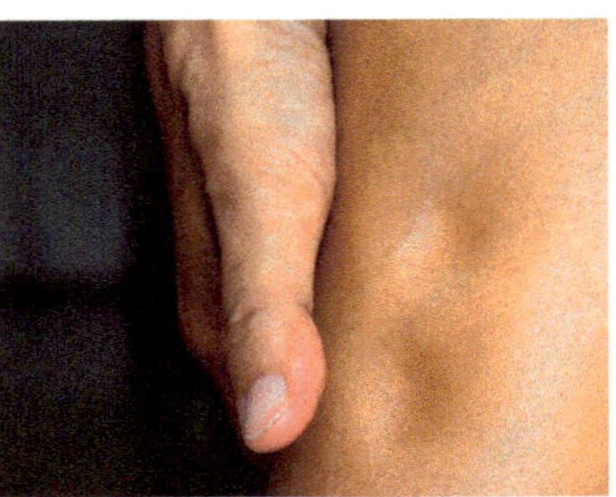
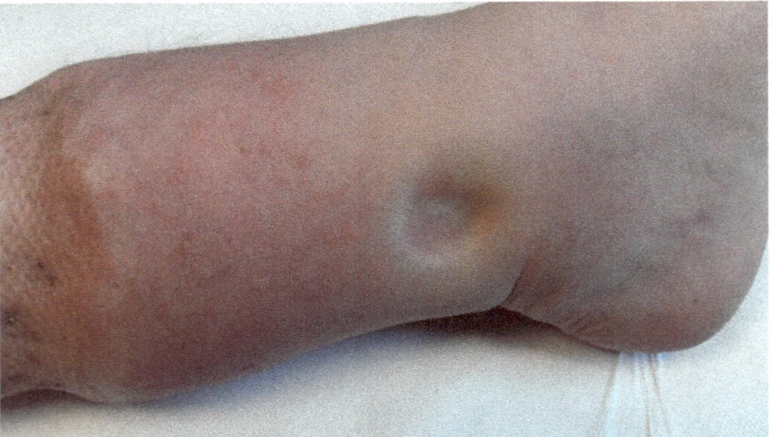

Figure 4.13   Example of a stage I lymphedema. Note the positive pitting sign. The actual pitting test is performed by applying pressure on the edema for at least 20 sec with one finger. The deeper the indentation, the more water is present. A deep indentation means that significant edema reduction can be achieved during therapy.

4.4.3　Stage II

Stage II edema can be defined as:

- Limb elevation alone rarely reduces tissue swelling and pitting is manifest.
- Late in stage II, the limb may or may not pit as excess fat and fibrosis supervenes. (Pitting becomes less and less prominent due to tissue formation).

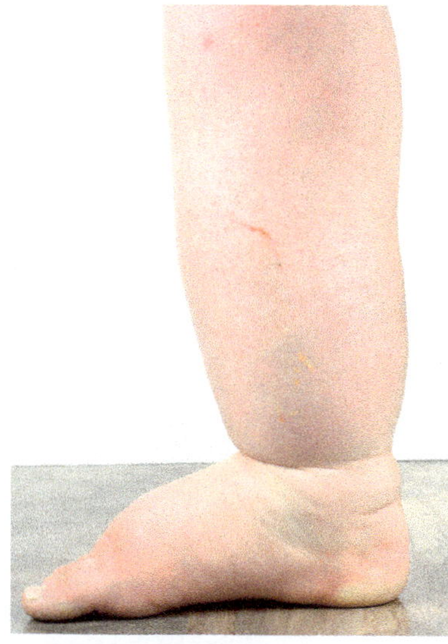
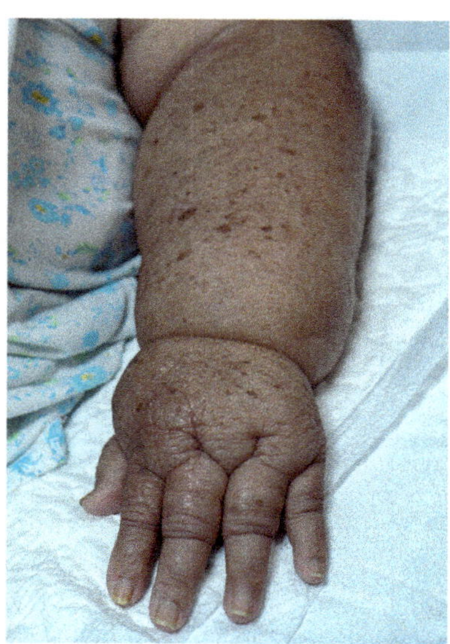
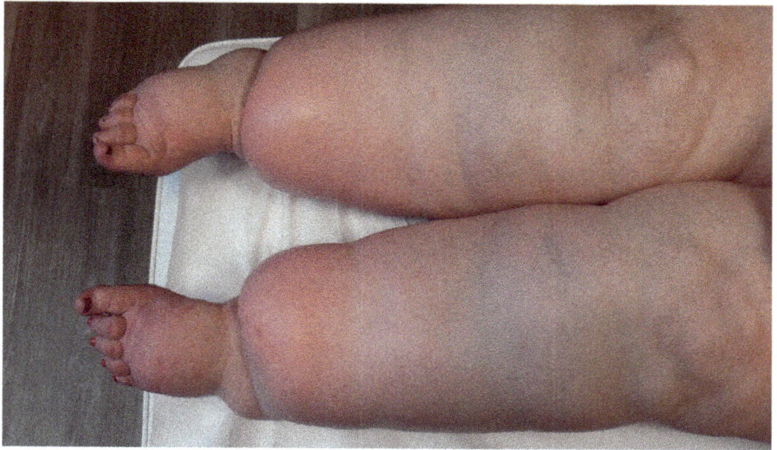

Figure 4.14　Examples of a stage II edema.

Note that stage II edema is often divided in IIa and IIb. IIa is characterized by pitting and tissue formation. In IIb, pitting is less obvious and tissue formation is predominant.

4.4.4   Stage III

Stage III edema encompasses lymphostatic elephantiasis, where pitting can be absent and trophic skin changes, such as acanthosis, further deposition of fat and fibrosis, and warty overgrowths have developed.

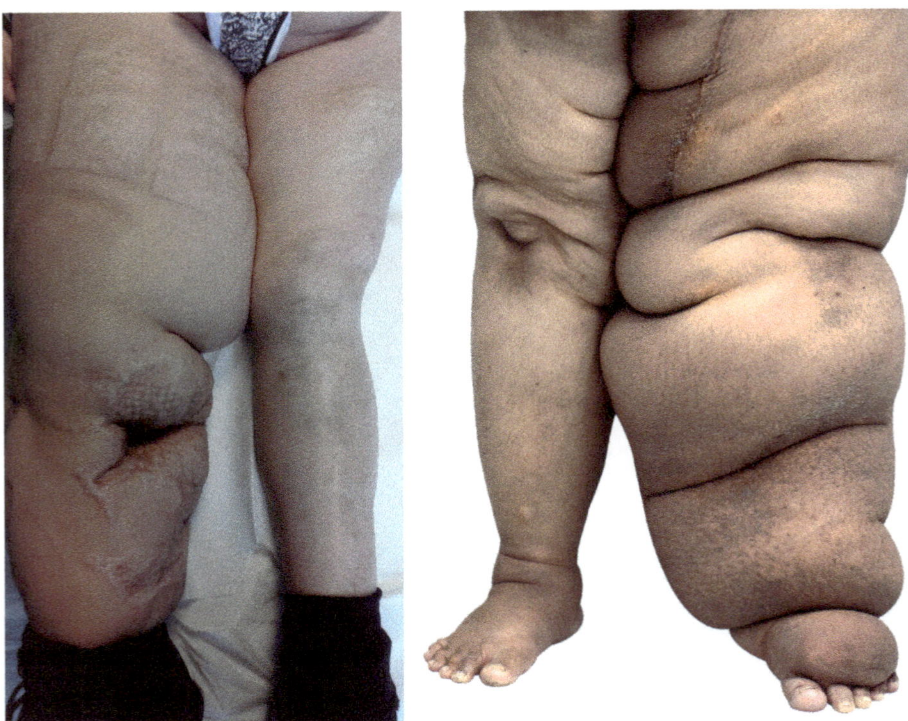

Figure 4.15   Stage III lymphedema with no pitting, skin changes and tissue formation.

Skin deformations, if present, are more likely to be present in late stage II and stage III of chronic edema. Apart from dry skin, thickened toenails also occur (as shown in figure 4.16).

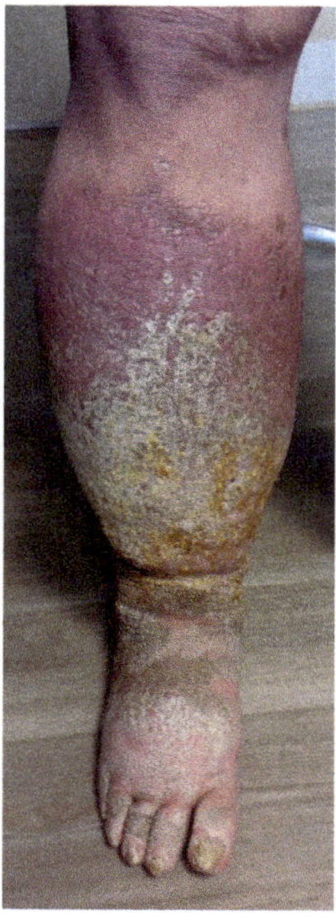

Figure 4.16   Example of a patient with lymphedema, dry kin, skin changes and trophic alterations of the toe nails.

This can also be seen in other conditions like eczema and fungal infections. Some specific skin deformations are seen in chronic edema:

- verrucosis, defined as a skin that looks like it has multiple warts;
- papillomatosis, the growth of different papilloma on the skin, which also look like warts.

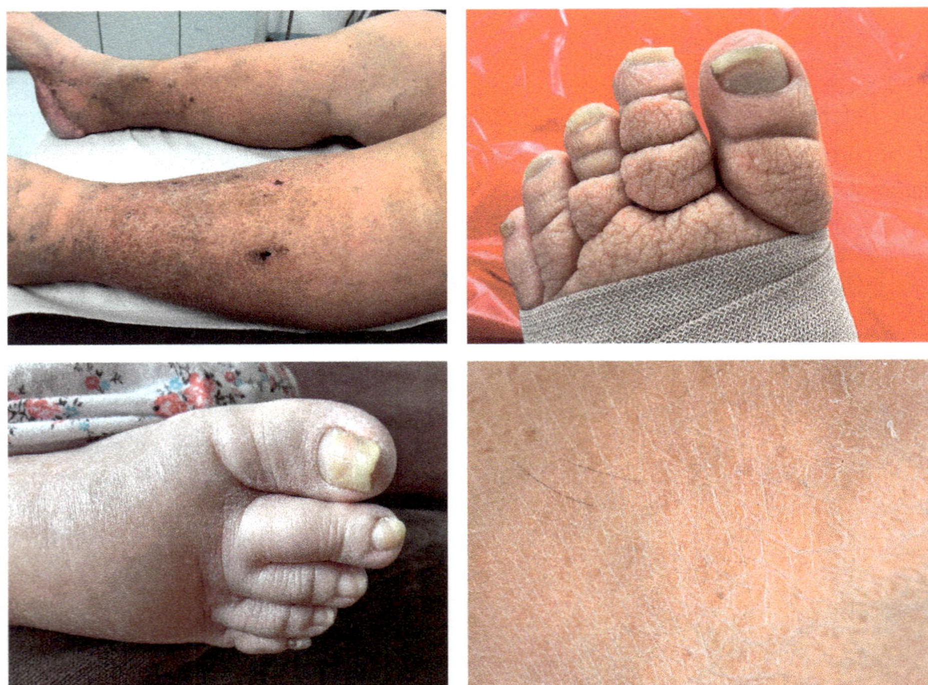

Figure 4.17 Some examples of specific skin deformations. Top, left to right: hyperpigmentation, changing toe nail. Bottom, left to right: damaged nails and skin, dry skin.

What the physiotherapist needs to know:
- In normal/healthy physiology there is only net filtration from the capillary towards the interstitial area in tissues like the skin, subcutis and muscle.
- Reabsorption through a capillary wall is only seen in specialized tissues like intestines or kidneys.
- The excess of interstitial fluid needs to be evacuated by the lymphatic system.
- Edema is only a symptom of disease, never the diagnosis as such.
- Pre-loading edema is provoked by excess fluid production from the microcirculation; the lymphatic system is working properly, yet unable to transport all excess fluid.
- After-loading edema is provoked by a failing lymphatic system.
- Both pre- and after-loading edema can coexist in a patient (e.g., CVI in combination with secondary lymphedema).

What other health-care workers need to know:

- In normal/healthy physiology there is only net filtration from the capillary towards the interstitial area in tissues like the skin, subcutis and muscle.
- Reabsorption through a capillary wall is only seen in specialized tissues like intestines or kidneys.
- There is no reabsorption in the capillary bed of most tissues like muscle, subcutis, cutis, and connective tissue.
- The lymphatic system is key in fluid transport from the interstitial area.
- There are a broad series of aetiologies that can cause chronic edema. Before starting therapy, a thorough work-up should be done to define its cause. If a treatable cause is found, then the appropriate treatment should be provided.
- Given the broad range of aetiologies of chronic edema, a multidisciplinary approach is warranted for the best diagnostic work-up.

4.5   REFERENCES

1. Wiig H, Swartz MA. Interstitial fluid and lymph formation and transport: physiological regulation and roles in inflammation and cancer. Physiol Rev. 2012;92(3):1005-1060.
2. Levick JR, Michel CC. Microvascular fluid exchange and the revised Starling principle. Cardiovasc Res. 2010;87(2):198-210.
3. Keast DH, Moffatt C, Janmohammad A. Lymphedema Impact and Prevalence International Study: The Canadian Data. Lymphat Res Biol. 2019;17(2):178-186.
4. Keeley V, Franks P, Quere I, et al. LIMPRINT in Specialist Lymphedema Services in United Kingdom, France, Italy, and Turkey. Lymphat Res Biol. 2019;17(2):141-146.
5. Moffatt C, Keeley V, Quere I. The Concept of Chronic Edema-A Neglected Public Health Issue and an International Response: The LIMPRINT Study. Lymphat Res Biol. 2019;17(2):121-126.
6. Quéré I, Palmier S, Noerregaard S, et al. LIMPRINT: Estimation of the Prevalence of Lymphoedema/Chronic Oedema in Acute Hospital in In-Patients. Lymphat Res Biol. 2019;17(2):135-140.
7. Damstra RJ, van Steensel MA, Boomsma JH, Nelemans P, Veraart JC. Erysipelas as a sign of subclinical primary lymphoedema: a prospective quantitative scintigraphic study of 40 patients with unilateral erysipelas of the leg. Br J Dermatol. 2008;158(6):1210-1215.
8. The diagnosis and treatment of peripheral lymphedema: 2020 Consensus Document of the International Society of Lymphology. Lymphology. 2020;53(1):3-19.

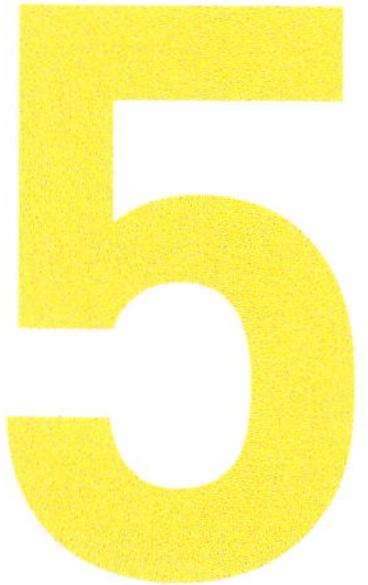

5 PREVENTION OF CHRONIC EDEMA

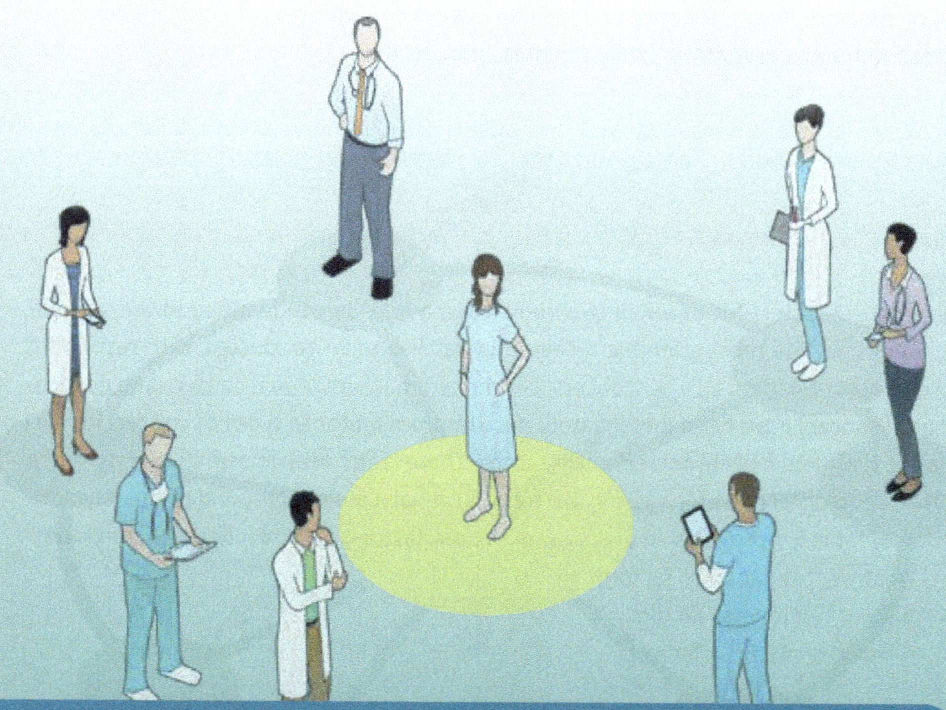

The learning objectives for this chapter are:
- Learning to identify patients at risk of developing chronic edema
- Providing insight into the decision-making process for patients at risk of developing chronic edema
- Providing insight into the preventive management for patients at risk of developing chronic edema

5.1 INTRODUCTION

Lymphedema or chronic edema is a chronic condition which can negatively impact a patient's physical and psychosocial health, in addition to his/her quality of life (QoL). It is therefore greatly important to set up clear instructions and guidelines for patients and health-care workers in the context of the preventive management of chronic edema. It has been shown that a healthy lifestyle has numerous benefits in the biopsychosocial context. Physical activity, a healthy body weight and a balanced diet can contribute to this healthy lifestyle and are beneficial to everyone, including lymphedema patients or patients at risk for lymphedema.

Firstly, it is necessary to identify patients at risk for developing chronic edema. Secondly, an assessment is necessary to determine whether early signs of chronic edema are present. If not, preventive management is appropriate.

5.2 IDENTIFICATION OF AT-RISK PATIENTS

Several risk factors for developing chronic edema have been identified in the scientific literature. The most scientific research by far has been conducted with respect to breast cancer patients. Other cancers, like melanomas, urogenital cancers and gynecological cancers have been investigated, but literature on those types of cancers in relation to risk factors of chronic edema is scarce. There is also little information concerning other aetiologies of lymphedema, like trauma, venous pathologies and primary lymphedema. Table 5.1 provides an overview of the risk factors, divided into three categories:

- treatment-related risk factors;
- patient-related risk factors;
- disease-related risk factors.

Treatment-related risk factors	
UPPER LIMB LYMPHEDEMA	LOWER LIMB LYMPHEDEMA
<ul><li>Axillary lymph node dissection compared to SLNB</li><li>Large number of lymph nodes dissected</li><li>Mastectomy compared to BCS</li><li>Cross over between ARM and SLN</li><li>Radiotherapy</li><li>Chemotherapy</li></ul>	<ul><li>Inguinal lymph node dissection compared to SLNB</li><li>Radiotherapy</li></ul>

Patient-related risk factors	
UPPER LIMB LYMPHEDEMA	LOWER LIMB LYMPHEDEMA
• Obesity • Large postoperative weight fluctuations • Not participating in regular physical activity	• Obesity
Disease-related risk factors	
UPPER LIMB LYMPHEDEMA	LOWER LIMP LYMPHEDEMA
• Metastatic lymph nodes • Advanced stage	• Advanced stage

Abbreviations: SLNB = sentinel lymph node biopsy, ARM = axillary reverse mapping, BCS = breast conserving surgery

Table 5.1   Identification of patients at risk.[1-3]

It is clear that a more invasive surgical (cancer) treatment poses a greater risk of developing chronic edema, especially when surgery is done in an area with a great number of lymph nodes (groin, pelvis, abdomen, axilla, neck). Yet the risk of developing chronic edema is present even in patients who undergo a more conservative approach like a SLNB or BCS, so it is very difficult to predict who will develop chronic edema. Also, it is likely that pre-existing factors, like underlying abnormalities in the lymphatic system and its drainage, can partly determine which patients will develop chronic edema and which will not.[2,4] In addition, the timing of when chronic edema will possibly occur cannot be predicted. The incidence of chronic edema is greater in the first two years after the oncological treatment. Of all patients who develop chronic edema, it occurs in 80% within two years after diagnosis and in 89% within three years.[5] Nevertheless, it is still possible to develop chronic edema several years after the initial cancer treatment.[6]

Since chronic edema and its timing are difficult to predict, it is recommended that all cancer patients whose lymphatic system could be potentially damaged be monitored systematically throughout their entire treatment and during follow-up. This should be done not only for patients who have undergone the more invasive lymph node dissection in the axilla or groin, but also for patients who received more conservative treatment.

After determining the patients at risk, an assessment is necessary to evaluate whether there are signs of swelling (see Chapter 6). Now, two options are possible:

- If, based on this assessment, signs of chronic edema are present, it is sometimes necessary to conduct a more thorough evaluation. These patients will also need to receive complex physical therapy (CPT) to properly treat their lymphedema (see Chapter 7).
- In patients who have no signs of swelling, preventive care is the appropriate approach.

5.3 PREVENTIVE MANAGEMENT FOR PATIENTS AT RISK

5.3.1 Monitoring for the onset of chronic edema

The literature shows that less severe lymphedema is easier to treat than severe lymphedema and has a better outcome.[7,8] The early detection of chronic edema is therefore of great importance. This can be done either by health- care workers or by the patient himself/herself (by means of a diary). For a detailed description of the assessment of chronic edema, see Chapter 6.

It is recommended that the limbs of patients be measured regularly during and after their cancer treatment. This can be done by a physiotherapist, breast nurse or medical doctor. Make sure the limbs are measured bilaterally in order to compare left to right. It is preferable to measure the limbs before surgery, during the after treatment and periodically during routine follow-up. If, during some time in this process, signs of chronic edema emerge, the patient should be referred to a specialized physiotherapist for appropriate treatment. Weekly self-assessment in which both limbs are measured at a fixed time during the day, together with a body weight measurement is a feasible approach. The patient can keep track of his/her records by keeping a diary.

In addition, it is valuable for patients to learn how to monitor themselves and recognize symptoms of chronic edema themselves. If a patient recognizes symptoms of heaviness, a feeling of swelling, tensed skin, clothing or jewelry that pinches and/or a print from clothing in the skin, they should seek medical help. The health-care worker to whom the patient is referred can perform a thorough check-up and recommend treatment, if necessary.

5.3.2 Skin care

The human skin forms an excellent barrier to infections. In patients at risk of developing chronic edema, the main purpose of skin care is to maintain that barrier by means of proper skin care. In Western countries, wounds, cellulitis and erysipelas are the most common causes of chronic edema related to infection. The literature shows that an infection can trigger a subclinical pre-existing lymphatic impairment, causing chronic edema.[4] It can also aggravate existing chronic edema. Meticulous skin care and skin hygiene is therefore mandatory in both the preventive and curative treatment for chronic edema. A detailed description of the skin care recommendations is provided in detail in Chapter 7.

5.3.3   Weight control

As mentioned above, overweight and obesity are risk factors for developing chronic edema. The link between overweight/obesity and the risk of developing chronic edema is the additional fluid shift provoked by the excess fat tissue. Fat cells also produce a hydrophilic substance that further increases the fluid shift.

Patients are advised to strive for optimal body weight. This means that they should maintain a normal body weight as much as possible or, in case of overweight or obese patients, to reduce their body weight. If necessary, it can be useful to work with a dietician and physical therapist or personal coach to implement exercise programmes that focus on weight loss.[2]

5.3.4   Exercises

Physical activity has numerous benefits related to our lymphatic system and lymphatic drainage. This is elaborated on in Chapter 7, which discusses the treatment of chronic edema. Furthermore, its health benefits in general are unmistakable, from muscle strength and muscle endurance to cardiovascular benefits.

Exercise therapy as part of the prevention of chronic edema involves a combination of active exercises of the limb in combination with breathing exercises. This stimulates the lymphatic transport by muscle pump activation and through the movement of the diaphragm and it stimulates lymphangiogenesis, which is the formation of new lymphatic vessels from pre-existing lymphatics. In addition to the effect on the lymphatic system, exercises are also beneficial with respect to arm and shoulder complaints in breast cancer patients, scars, fatigue and other morbidities related to cancer treatment (see Chapter 2).

As mentioned previously, patients who are not physically active are at greater risk of developing chronic edema. Therefore, after their cancer treatment, it is recommended that at-risk patients resume at least the same level of physical activity as they had before. Many patients have a tendency to spare their limb(s) after surgery, although there is strong evidence that physical activity, even strenuous activities, are safe to execute without increasing the risk of chronic edema. It is the physiotherapist's job to reassure the patients that physical activity is completely safe and has many benefits, and to coach the patient into finding an activity which he or she finds comfortable, such as walking, cycling and swimming.[2]

The most important findings from the literature are displayed in table 5.2. Scientific evidence concerning the preventive effect of exercises on chronic edema in the lower limbs is currently lacking.

Author, journal, year	Study design	Conclusion
Box et al., Breast Cancer Res Treat, 2002[9]	RCT	A combination of monitoring, information and exercises are effective in the prevention of BCRL
Schmitz et al., JAMA, 2010[10]	RCT	Exercises (weightlifting) are effective in the prevention of BCRL
Cheema et al., Breast Cancer Res Treat, 2008[11]	Systematic review of 10 studies	No patient developed arm edema after a period of progressive resistance training

Table 5.2 Scientific evidence concerning the preventive effect of exercises on lymphedema.

5.3.5   What about manual lymphatic drainage?

The effectiveness of manual lymphatic drainage (MLD) as part of the prevention of chronic edema is currently still up for debate. The most important findings from the literature are displayed in table 5.3. All three studies are included in the meta-analysis of Stuiver et al.[12] Scientific evidence concerning the preventive effect of exercises on chronic edema in the lower limbs is currently lacking.

Author, journal, year	Study design	Conclusion
Torres Lacomba et al., BMJ, 2010[13]	RCT	MLD in combination with exercises is effective in the prevention of BCRL
Zimmermann et al., Lymphology, 2012[14]	RCT	MLD is effective in the prevention of BCRL
Devoogdt et al., BMJ, 2011[15]	RCT	MLD has no preventive effect on the development of BCRL in the short and long term.

Table 5.3 Scientific evidence concerning the preventive effect of MLD on lymphedema.

As seen in table 5.3, several studies found contradicting results. Therefore, no firm conclusions can be drawn about the added value of MLD in addition to monitoring, skin care, weight control and exercises. Nevertheless, it is our recommendation to withdraw MLD from the preventive treatment of chronic edema due to the lack of strong scientific evidence, together with the fact that it is time-consuming and costly.

What the physiotherapist needs to know:

- All cancer patients in whom the lymphatic system could be potentially damaged have to be considered as at-risk patients for the development of chronic edema.
- Monitor patients consistently by assessing the limbs bilaterally. In addition, teach the patients to recognize symptoms of chronic edema himself/herself.
- The prevention of chronic edema consists of monitoring, skin care, weight control and exercises.
- Preventive MLD has no added value.
- If the patient shows signs of chronic edema, start the complex decongestive treatment.

What other health-care workers need to know:

- Risk patients should be monitored closely, preferably prior to their cancer treatment, during the treatment and periodically during follow-up.
- If signs of chronic edema are present, refer the patient to a specialized physiotherapist for appropriate treatment.

5.4   REFERENCES

1. Gebruers N, Verbelen H, De Vrieze T, et al. Current and future perspectives on the evaluation, prevention and conservative management of breast cancer related lymphoedema: A best practice guideline. Eur J Obstet Gynecol Reprod Biol. 2017;216:245-253. doi:10.1016/j.ejogrb.2017.07.035
2. The Dutch lymphedema guidelines based on the International Classification of Functioning, Disability, and Health and the chronic care model. Damstra RJ, Halk AB; Dutch Working Group on Lymphedema. J Vasc Surg Venous Lymphat Disord. 2017;5(5):756-765. doi: 10.1016/j.jvsv.2017.04.012.
3. DiSipio T, Rye S, Newman B, Hayes S. Incidence of unilateral arm lymphoedema after breast cancer: A systematic review and meta-analysis. Lancet Oncol. 2013;14(6):500-515. doi:10.1016/S1470-2045(13)70076-7
4. Damstra RJ, Van Steensel MAM, Boomsma JHB, Nelemans P, Veraart JCJM. Erysipelas as a sign of subclinical primary lymphoedema: A prospective quantitative scintigraphic study of 40 patients with unilateral erysipelas of the leg. Br J Dermatol. 2008;158(6):1210-1215. doi:10.1111/j.1365-2133.2008.08503.x
5. Norman SA, Localio AR, Potashnik SL, et al. Lymphedema in Breast Cancer Survivors: Incidence, Degree, Time Course, Treatment, and Symptoms. J Clin Oncol. 2008;27:390-397. doi:10.1200/JCO.2008.17.9291

6. Clark B, Sitzia J, Harlow W. Incidence and risk of arm oedema following treatment for breast cancer: A three-year follow-up study. QJM. 2005;98(5):343-348. doi:10.1093/qjmed/hci053

7. Johansson K, Branje E. Arm lymphoedema in a cohort of breast cancer survivors 10 years after diagnosis. Acta Oncol. 2010;49(2):166-173. doi:10.3109/02841860903483676

8. Mcneely ML, Magee DJ, Lees AW, Bagnall KM, Haykowsky M, Hanson J. The Addition of Manual Lymph Drainage to Compression Therapy for Breast Cancer Related Lymphedema: A Randomized Controlled Trial. Breast Cancer Res Treat. 2004 Jul;86(2):95-106. doi: 10.1023/B:BREA.0000032978.67677.9f.

9. Box RC, Reul-Hirche HM, Bullock-Saxton JE, Furnival CM. Physiotherapy after Breast Cancer Surgery: Results of a Randomised Controlled Study to Minimise Lymphoedema. Breast Cancer Res Treat. 2002 Sep;75(1):51-64. doi: 10.1023/a:1016591121762.

10. 10.Schmitz KH. Balancing Lymphedema Risk. Exerc Sport Sci Rev. 2010;38(1):17-24. doi:10.1097/JES.0b013e3181c5cd5a

11. Cheema B, Gaul CA, Lane K, Fiatarone Singh MA. Progressive resistance training in breast cancer: a systematic review of clinical trials. Breast Cancer Res Treat. 2008 May;109(1):9-26. doi: 10.1007/s10549-007-9638-0.

12. Stuiver MM, ten Tusscher MR, Agasi-Idenburg CS, Lucas C, Aaronson NK, Bossuyt PM. Conservative interventions for preventing clinically detectable upper-limb lymphoedema in patients who are at risk of developing lymphoedema after breast cancer therapy. Cochrane Database Syst Rev. 2015;13;(2):CD009765. doi: 10.1002/14651858.CD009765.

13. Lacomba MT, Sánchez MJY, Goñi ÁZ, et al. Effectiveness of early physiotherapy to prevent lymphoedema after surgery for breast cancer: Randomised, single blinded, clinical trial. BMJ. 2010;340(7738):140. doi:10.1136/bmj.b5396

14. Zimmermann A, Wozniewski M, Szklarska A, Lipowicz A, Szuba A. Efficacy of manual lymphatic drainage in preventing secondary lymphedema after breast cancer surgery. Lymphology. 2012 Sep;45(3):103-12. PMID: 23342930.

15. Devoogdt N, Christiaens M-R, Geraerts I, et al. Effect of manual lymph drainage in addition to guidelines and exercise therapy on arm lymphoedema related to breast cancer: randomised controlled trial. BMJ. 2011;343:d5326. doi:10.1136/bmj.d5326

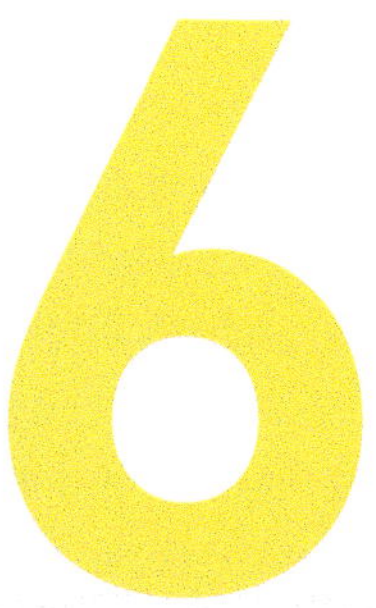

6 PHYSICAL EXAMINA-TION AND CLINICAL ASSESSMENT

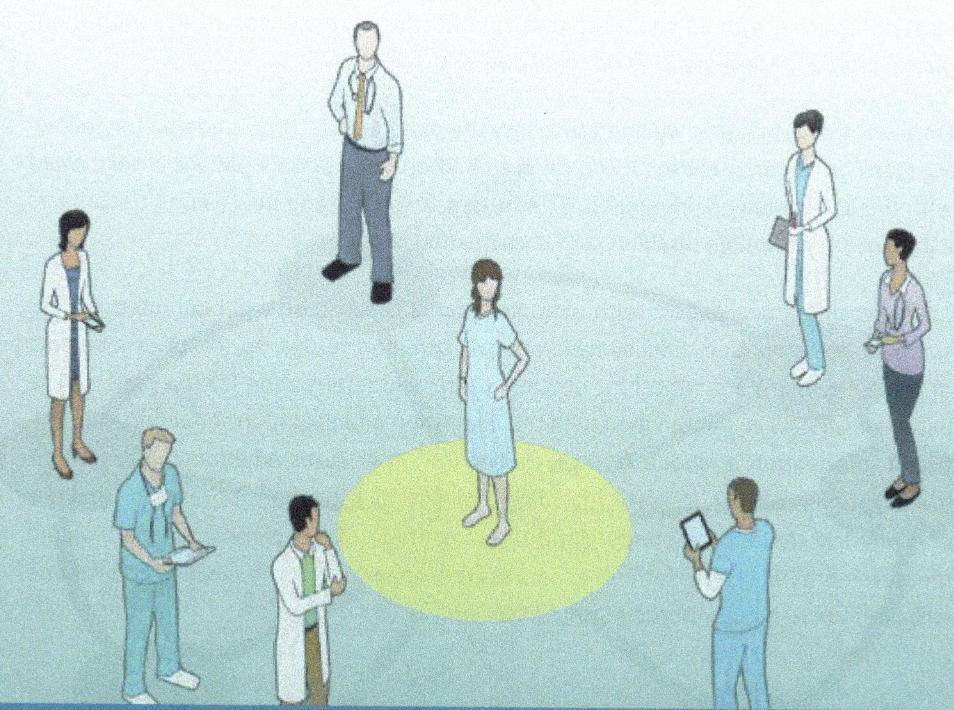

The learning objectives for this chapter are:
- Providing a comprehensive structure that can be used for the clinical examination of patients with chronic edema
- Providing background knowledge on the technical investigations that are most commonly used in patients with chronic edema with the purpose of educating and informing the patients
- Providing evidence-based approaches for the assessment of the edema volume as well as other investigation or questionnaire to capture the full extent of chronic edema in an ICF model

6.1　INTRODUCTION

This chapter should be read with the following assumptions in mind. First, it is assumed that the patient has been referred with the existence of swelling. For monitoring at-risk patients and preventive management, see Chapter 5. The methods of assessment of a patient with chronic edema are further explained in this chapter. Second, all effort should be made to rule out any treatable causes like hormone disturbances, kidney failure, heart failure or medication interactions that could provoke the edema. Third, if by exclusion of the different differential diagnoses the diagnosis of a chronic edema is made, then an investigation of the vascular system (often done by a vascular surgeon) should confirm a normal ankle brachial index or ABI (should be at least 0.9; if the ABI = 0.8 or lower, the compression therapy should be adjusted to the ABI) to ensure the safety of starting with edema treatment. In other words, thrombosis and serious peripheral arterial disease need to be ruled out.

Once we are certain that we need to assess the patient with chronic edema the following steps are recommended. A clinical examination of an edema patient is performed with the ICF framework in mind. It is important to understand how a condition affects a patient's functioning, disability and participation in society.

The assessment of a patient with (chronic) edema is based on a patient interview, inspection and palpation. Clinical tests are less common to use, so the prior elements of the assessment are critical for obtaining sufficient information from a patient. The patient interview in combination with the inspection and palpation should provide sufficient information in about 7/10 cases. For the other cases additional information/investigation is often necessary, including technical investigations beyond the abilities of a physical therapist. To understand the magnitude of the chronic edema, volume measurements will be performed to address the magnitude of the swelling and volume will continue to be monitored during follow-up.

6.2　PATIENT INTERVIEW

A patient's interview is a key component and should be done thoroughly.[1,2] After the inventory of the referral and collecting the necessary patient data, the actual interview can start.

Key elements that need to be discussed are:
- The patient's request for help: what does the patient want to achieve? It is very important to listen to the patient's request and not only what the physician has men-

tioned during the referral. What are the perspectives mentioned by the patient? What are the barriers mentioned by the patient? It is very important to discuss any misconceptions or unrealistic goals; if any are present, take sufficient time to dispel them and present a more realistic picture. Next, it is important to state that lifelong management is necessary in many cases and that a return to normalcy is seldom achievable. In other words, listen very carefully but do not give patients false hope. Sometimes patients have consulted the internet in search of answers, and we all know that Dr. Google is not always right.

- **The current complaint's timeline, its onset and 24-hour alterations:** try to get a detailed idea of the first onset of the problem. For patients with chronic edema it is very common to have complaints for many months up to even years. It is important to understand whether or not there was a clear provocation of the complaints (primary versus secondary onset of edema). Discuss how the complaints have evolved over time (worsening or not). Discuss which types of treatment have already been tried out. Discuss 24-hour alterations. In early onset, you will expect to have alterations between day and night (awake hours versus sleeping hours). Most common edema complaints will increase as patients are awake and upright against gravity. If the edema is already long-lasting, the alterations during 24 hours will be less explicitly present and patients will report limited fluctuations in swelling but perhaps a more heavy and annoying sensation, even more painful as waking hours progress.

- **Comorbidity and prior treatment:** important comorbidities to rule out or discuss are heart disease, thyroid malfunction (especially hypothyroidism), kidney disease/function, low albumin, diabetes, infections, surgery and trauma. Ask about all the treatments and their outcomes that are ongoing or have been tried in the past.

- **Medication:** it is important to know what medication the patient is taking and its impact on circulatory physiology. It is especially important to know whether the patient is taking diuretics, corticosteroids or hormone substitution. If medication is supposed to be a contributing factor to the edema, you should consult the treating physician and discuss the possibilities for an altered medication scheme. In some patients it can result from the interaction between different types of medication; if suspected, consult the treating physician and discuss the options. Known interactions can be found in databases like UpToDate (uptodate.com).
You can find a link to the UpToDate calculators at the online learning platform Sofia.

- **Physical activities:** since physical activities have a beneficial effect during the treatment of edema, it is important to assess PA and its type, frequency and intensity. It is also important to find out whether the patient is motivated to engage in regular exercises or physical activity. Exercising is often a barrier to patients, especially in the maintenance phase when exercising is mostly unsupervised.

- **Technical investigations:** discuss which investigations already have been performed to objectify the edema. Important investigations are a blood sample to check hormone and protein (especially albumin) levels, a cardiac ultrasound (echocardiogram), lymphangiography, scintigraphy or other imaging techniques to qualitatively or quantitively assess the lymphatics and/or blood vessels.

- the interview should assess prior severe viral or bacterial infections, (e.g., Epstein-Barr, Borrelia, Streptococcus, Staphylococcus), prior events of cellulitis or erysipelas, severe episodes of fever, trauma and prior surgery. If patients have had surgery, try to get details on the extent of surgery, likeliness of lymphatic damage (due to the area of surgery), presence of scars, radiation therapy, chemotherapy, etc. Also ask about recent travels to (sub-tropical) countries to rule out a possible parasite infection.
- Family history: the interview should include questions regarding the presence of syndromes in the family and the presence of edema in other family members.
- ICF-inventory: use the ICF framework to ascertain the impact of the current complaints on ADL/ QoL/ functioning and participation in society. This item can perfectly be assessed by means of questionnaires like the Lymph-ICF-UL or Lymph-ICF-LL. These questionnaires provide information on five different ICF domains. For a detailed description of these questionnaires, see the article *Lymphoedema Functioning, Disability and Health Questionnaire for Lower Limb Lymphoedema (Lymph-ICF-LL): Reliability and Validity*. You can also read a *Revision of the Lymphedema Functioning, Disability and Health Questionnaire for Upper Limb Lymphedema (Lymph-ICF-UL): Reliability and validity.*
A link to these articles is provided on the online learning platform Sofia.

6.3   INSPECTION

The inspection, together with the palpation, can generate important information about the cause as well as the impact and distribution of the edema.[1-3] Always inspect the patient as a whole, not only the edema area. Use the umbilicus as a point of reference. In edema of the legs, inspect the patient up to the height of the umbilicus. For the upper body, start at the umbilicus and inspect further upwards. The key elements during inspection are:

- Distribution of the edema: check if it is possible to define a strict border of the edema. Define whether it is a one-sided, bilateral or midline edema (head, trunk, genitalia).
- Trophic changes: trophic changes are changes to the skin, nails and hair growth. The skin can either appear shiny when there is a lot of tension in the skin due to accumulation of fluid underneath it (often seen in early stage edema or in fast progressive edema). Another appearance of the skin is dryness and flakiness. You will see skin that is covered in white skin flakes. In severe and long-lasting edema, skin

changes such as papillomatosis or verrucosis can be seen (see Chapter 4). Nails tend to thicken and become dull and yellow and fragile. Most commonly, hair growth disappears over the edematous area.

- Colour: different colours can be seen:
  - pale/white: dry skin, uncomplicated lymphedema, due to the presence of peripheral arterial disease;
  - red: arterial problem like DVT, phlebitis, inflammation, infections;
  - brown: ferritin deposits due to chronic venous disorder, melanoma, hyperpigmentation, (radio)dermatitis;
  - blue/cyanotic: venous pooling, cyanosis, hematoma.
- Scars/wounds: check the edematous area and its surrounding for the presence of scars and wounds. Scars can provide information about trauma or surgery. Wounds will tend to heal slowly and badly on an edematous area without any additional care.
- Footwear and/or possible compression material: check to see whether the patient wears appropriate footwear that doesn't pinch, in order to secure the lymphatic drainage through the muscle pump and to prevent blisters or wounds on toes or feet. Also, if patients are wearing compression garments, check to make sure that they don't pinch either and check whether the fit and height of the compression garment is appropriate.

6.4   PALPATION

There are actually no tests for assessing the functionality of the lymphatic system that can be used in the examination of patients with chronic edema. It is therefore important to use the following palpatory tests to gain additional information about the type and extent of the edema.[2]

- Pitting sign: the pitting test is performed by applying firm pressure to an edematous area. The pressure is sustained for at least 20 seconds (original study stated 1 minute). If afterwards an indentation is visible or palpable, this is a positive pitting sign. A positive pitting sign confirms that the swelling is mainly fluid. The deeper the indentation, the more excess fluid within the interstitial space. If the indentation is limited or even absent, tissue formation is present. Tissue formation is seen in the later stages of lymphedema. Once tissue formation is present, a limited reduction of the edema volume can be achieved with the conservative decongestive treatment. It is therefore important that patients do not wait too long to consult a physician. If there is a significant and disproportional edema volume the patient might be a candidate for lymphosuction surgery. It has been demonstrated that the pitting signs correlate with lymphatic pathology in a sample of BCRL patients.[4]

- the stemmer test is performed by picking up a skinfold at the base of the second toe or second finger. Since edema is a combination of fluid and proteins, skinfolds will thicken over time, resulting in tissue formation. The results of the stemmer test are:
  - normal skinfold;
  - abnormal skinfold but still possible to pick up a skinfold;
  - unable to pick up a skin fold.

  The stemmer test provides information regarding the extent to which tissue formation is already present in the edematous limb.
- Pinching test: the pinching test is performed by pinching the skin. If edema is present it will be impossible to wrinkle the skin; without edema the skin will wrinkle. This test is performed to determine the extent and location of the edema.[4]
- Capillary refill test (CRT): the CRT is executed by applyiing pressure to a toe- or fingernail until the nail turns white. Upon releasing the pressure, the seconds are counted until the colour normalizes. Under normal conditions, normal colour is reached within 3 seconds. If the test is abnormal it is still inconclusive, as several different reasons could be responsible for the positive CRT. For instance, peripheral arterial disease (PAD) or heart failure or dehydration will all result in a positive CRT, warranting further investigations when CRT is abnormal. (The CRT is also a test that should be performed after the application of a compression bandage to test arterial flow).

6.5 TECHNICAL EXAMINATIONS AND EDEMA ASSESSMENT

As mentioned above, the patient interview in combination with the questionnaires, inspection and palpatory tests are critical for obtaining essential information. In many cases this information will be sufficient to start therapy; however, in some cases additional (technical) investigations are warranted. If no additional investigations are needed, you can proceed with the edema assessment.

Next, a brief description of the most common technical examinations will be provided. This information can be used to understand the aim and execution of these investigations. It can also serve as information to share with a patient. In this way the patient is better informed and more able to understand the importance of the investigation regarding the current problem.

After the technical investigations, we will elaborate on the different assessments used to obtain information regarding the edema volume. This type of assessment will be done by the PT and is often requested by the health insurance company in connection with the reimbursement of the treatment for chronic edema.

6.5.1   Technical examinations

6.5.1.1   Lymphoscintigraphy

A lymphoscintigraphy is a special investigation that needs to be performed by nuclear physicians in a hospital setting.[5] Lymphoscintigraphy assesses the body's lymphatic system using small amounts of radioactive materials (called radiotracers) bound to large proteins (e.g., albumin) that are typically injected into the skin. The radiotracer travels through the area being examined (lymphatic system) and the energy in the form of gamma rays is detected by a special gamma camera. A computer with imaging software will create images of the inside of your body. Because it is able to pinpoint molecular activity within the body, lymphoscintigraphy has the potential to identify lymphatic disease in its earliest stages.

The radiotracer will be injected just beneath the skin, or sometimes deeper, using a very small needle.

Most common lymphoscintigraphic investigation is called a 3-phase lymphoscintigraphy. This type of scintigraphy is also requested by the health insurance company, and as such it is very important that this investigation is executed properly and the report is written accordingly.

The three phases of a scintigraphy for the examination of the lymphatic system are:
- Phase 1: immediately after the injection, the gamma camera will take a series of images of the area of the body being studied.
- Phase 2: the patient performs an exercise for about 10 minutes (moving the feet or squeezing a soft ball between the fingers. If patients are unable to do exercises, the injection site is massaged). After exercising, another series of images are taken.
- Phase 3: the patient is instructed to walk or to be physically active for about 1 hour. After this, a third series of images are taken. After completion of the examination the results are written into a report with regard to minor and major criteria. Minor criteria refer to a decreased uptake or flow within the lymphatic system, while major criteria refer to the absence of flow or incomplete flow with dermal backflow pattern. Dermal backflow refers to the pathological situation where the tracer extravasates from the lymphatic system, resulting in incomplete transport.

6.5.1.2 Doppler ultrasound

Ultrasound imaging is based on the same principles involved in the sonar used by bats, ships and fishermen. When a sound wave strikes an object, it bounces back, or echoes. By measuring these echo waves, it is possible to determine how far away the object is as well as the object's size, shape and consistency. This includes whether the object is solid or filled with fluid.

In medicine, ultrasound is used to detect changes in the appearance of organs, tissues and vessels and to detect abnormal masses, such as tumours.

In an ultrasound exam, a transducer both sends the sound waves and records the echoing waves. When the transducer is pressed against the skin, it sends small pulses of inaudible, high-frequency sound waves into the body. As the sound waves bounce off internal organs, fluids and tissues, the sensitive receiver in the transducer records tiny changes in the sound's pitch and direction. These signature waves are instantly measured and displayed by a computer, which in turn creates a real-time picture on the monitor. One or more frames of the moving pictures are typically captured as still images. Short video loops of the images may also be saved.

Doppler ultrasound is a special ultrasound technique that measures the direction and speed of blood cells flowing through vessels.[6] The movement of blood cells causes a change in pitch of the reflected sound waves (called the Doppler effect). A computer collects and processes the sounds and creates graphs or colour pictures that represent the flow of blood (unidirectional, increased flow, decreased flow) through the blood vessels. A venous sonogram is primarily used to diagnose deep vein thrombosis (DVT). Other reasons for a venous ultrasound may include:

- identifying the cause of leg swelling;
- locating damaged valves;
- aiding in certain medical procedures;
- blood clots;
- damaged or dysfunctional valves in the veins of your legs;
- defects of your heart valve(s);
- congenital heart disease;
- low blood circulation to your legs;
- aneurysms;
- peripheral arterial disease (PAD/PVD) → ABI assessment.

6.5.1.3 Lymphofluoroscopy

During a lymphofluoroscopy, a small dose of diluted Indocyanine Green (ICG) is injected intradermally in the first and fourth web space of the hand-fingers/foot-toes on the affected side. ICG emits fluorescence in the near-infrared spectrum (760 nm) and the signal is acquired using a camera with a Photo Dynamic Eye (PDE) system to visualize the superficial lymphatic system to a depth of maximum 20 mm.[7] The procedure consists of three consecutive phases, comparable to a 3-phase lymphoscintigraphy.

- During the first part of the investigation, lymph flow is evaluated at rest, after activity, and after stimulating lymph transport with MLD.
- Phase two consists of a 60 min break in which exercise and rest are alternated.
- Lastly, in phase three, a scan of the limb (upper or lower) is performed with the PDE camera.

During this real-time assessment by the PDE camera, pictures are taken, or video is recorded of the lymphatics.

Sometimes, functional lymph nodes together with active lymphatic transport as well as dysfunctional rerouting patterns are designed on a body diagram. All the information about the lymphatic transport is documented in a standard evaluation document.

During a lymphofluoroscopy, the superficial lymphatic network can be visualized. Since a fluoroscopy is a real-time investigation, an appreciation of the functionality of the lymphatic system can be made. The investigation itself is based upon the technology of near infrared imaging. By injecting ICG, a fluorescent substance that binds with albumin, a visualisation of the distribution of the ICG can be assessed. A fluoroscopy is supplemental to a scintigraphic investigation. A clear advantage of the fluoroscopy is that it provides real-time information about the routing of the lymph fluid. This information can aid the treatment of the lymphedema because therapists know the draining route.

Different pathologic situation can be demonstrated by means of lymphofluorsocopy. In figures 6.1-6.5 the different images are explained.

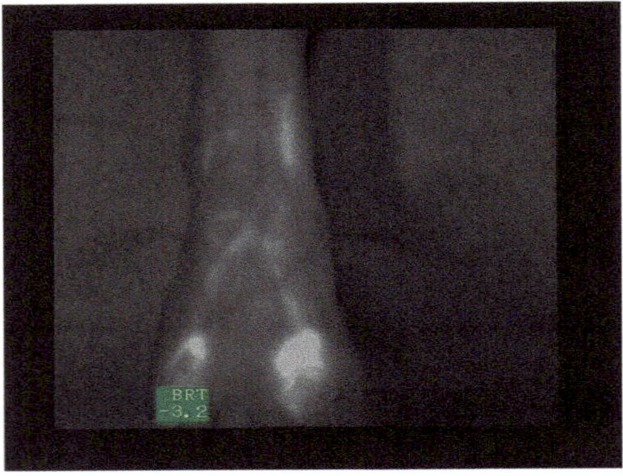

Figure 6.1   A normal linear pattern as seen in a healthy lymphatic system.

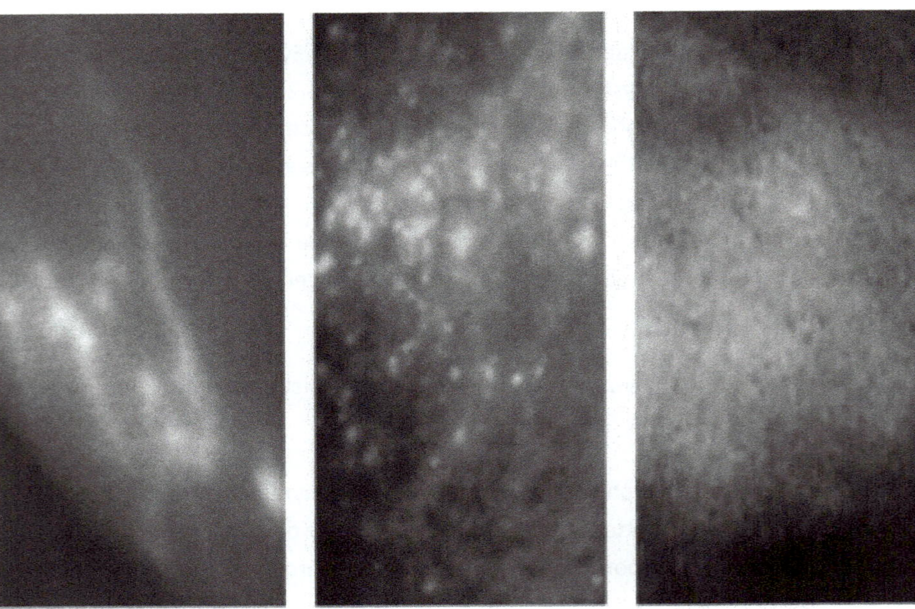

Figure 6.2   Abnormal lymphatic anatomy as seen by a lymphofluoroscopic investigation. From left to right: rerouting/splash, stardust and diffuse.

Rerouting/splash

Fluid in the initial lymphatics has difficulty progressing to the pre-collectors.

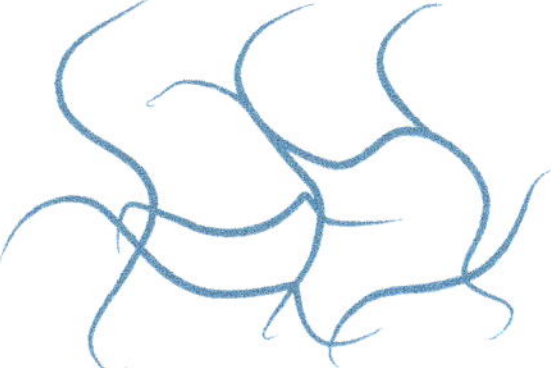

Figure 6.3   Rerouting/splash.

Stardust

Fluid remains in the pre-collectors without progressing into the collectors. The cross-section of the precollectors are visible.

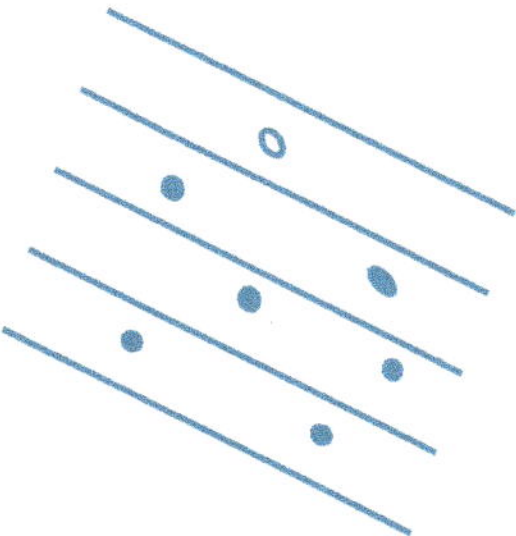

Figure 6.4   Stardust.

Diffuse

ICG is diluted into the interstitial fluid without any uptake by the lymphatic system.

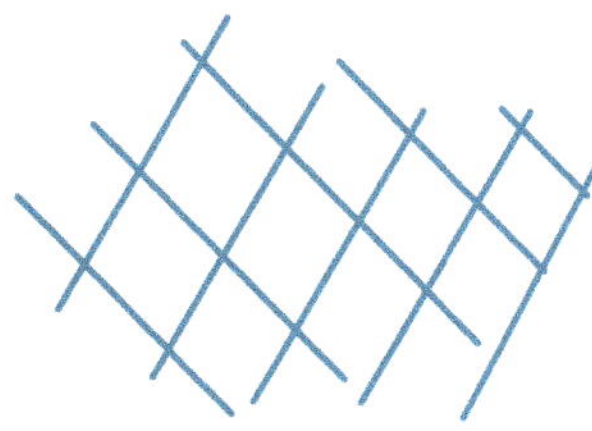

Figure 6.5   Diffuse.

Dermal backflow

Due to a blockage in a lymph collector, the lymph cannot move proximally in the lymph collector but drains through the precollectors and the lymph capillaries towards the interstitium. This is seen in lymphedema patients. Because of gravity, the lymph fluid in the interstitium often moves distally.

Dermal rerouting

Due to a blockage in a lymph collector, the lymph moves to the lymph capillaries and seeks a functional collector.

6.5.1.4 Other investigations:

MRI/CT/ genetic testing can be performed, as well. Most often these types of investigations are limited and only for selected patients in which aetiology is difficult to determine or a syndrome is suspected. When treating a patient as a PT and you are unable to get sufficient results, it can be worthwhile to contact the treating physician and discuss further diagnostic options before continuing treatment.

6.5.2 Edema assessment

In the following sections, edema assessments that can be used by the PT will be discussed.[8] Always inform yourself about the prevailing regulations of the health insurance company in order to select the most appropriate assessment for filing your report. Additionally, several assessments have been found valid and reliable in scientific research. Sometimes, new assessments were tested for the sole purpose of doing research. Therefore, some assessments are not readily available for clinical practice.

In the sections below we will focus on the assessments that have good clinimetric properties (read: are valid and reliable) and are readily available for PTs to use in clinical practice as well as for scientific research.

6.5.2.1 Water Displacement (gold standard)

Water displacement may be used to diagnose chronic edema. Different definitions have been used in the past, e.g., volume difference of more than 200 mL when compared with the contralateral arm or more than 10% interlimb difference.[9] This technique is often regarding as limited by clinical utility. The technique is found to be cumbersome due to the heavy weight once the volumeter has been filled with water. It has a hygienic aspect (having to change the water for every patient) and is time consuming (Evidence Quality: Level 1 reliability and validity; Level II diagnostic accuracy; Recommendation Strength: Grade B).[8-11] In clinical practice, the difference between both limbs is often defined as 0-5%, 5-10% and >10% difference. 0-5% is mostly referred to self-management with compression garments. 5-10% calls for intensive treatment with subsequently self-management and compression garments. >10 and >30% differences indicate severe lymphedema, which are treated with intensive treatment and treatment by additional disciplines (psychology, nutrition, dermatology). This is then followed by self-management with compression garments/exercise and self-massage.[1]

Alternative water displacement methods are available:
- The Valgrado system combines a volumeter, electronic scale and PC to assess the volume directly during the water displacement. Currently, this type of volumeter is not commercially available.
- In 2007 Gebruers et al. introduced prediction formulas based on normative data for arm volumes.[10] These prediction formulas enable the assessment of unilateral upper limb edema. The formulas are more strict in defining chronic edema than common definitions (e.g., 200ml, 10% volume difference[9]) as they consider handedness and gender (table 6.1).

Prediction statement	Prediction equation (± prediction interval)
Prediction of right arm volume of a right handed male	$= 0.995$ (vol. left arm) $+ 116.79$ ml (± 181.25 ml)
Prediction of left arm volume of a right handed male	$= 0.964$ (vol. right arm) $- 1,5$ ml (± 179.62 ml)
Prediction of right arm volume of a right handed female	$= 0.979$ (vol. left arm) $+ 96.66$ ml (± 148.66 ml)
Prediction of left arm volume of a right handed female	$= 0.991$ (vol. right arm) $- 33.33$ ml (± 148.10 ml)
Prediction of right arm volume of left handed males and females	$= 0.949$ (vol. left arm) $+ 88.66$ ml (± 227.69 ml)
Prediction of left arm volume of left handed males and females	$= 1.001$ (vol. right arm) $+ 43.97$ ml (± 234.22 ml)

Table 6.1 Evaluation of upper extremities in 250 healthy individuals.

To use this type of water displacement you will need an arm volumeter and electronic scale as demonstrated in figure 6.6. The procedure to obtain the volume of both arms is as follows. First, set up the volumeter and scale on a level surface and fill the volumeter with tepid water (28-32°C) until it overflows. Second, mark both arms of the patient at the mid-humerus level. The mid-humerus level is defined by ½ the distance between the lower margin of the acromion and the most prominent part of lateral epicondyle of the humerus. This distance can best be assessed with 90° of flexion in the elbow joint. Third, position the patient alongside the volumeter as close as possible to the volumeter. Confirm that the electronic scale is tarred with the recipient in place. Once in position the patient can submerse the first arm into the volumeter to the height of the mid-humerus marking. Wait until the water stops overflowing from the volumeter and write down the volume as the weight of the water is equal to the amount of ml (1g of water = 1ml of water). Fourth, refill the volumeter until it overflows again. Once calibrated the other arm can be assessed by repeating step three.

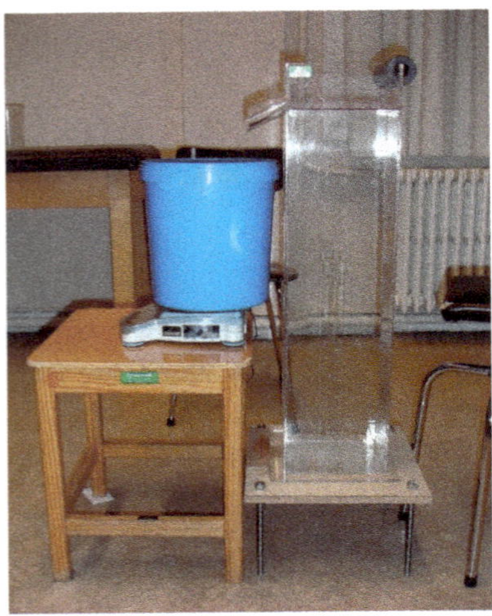

Figure 6.6 Setup of a commercially available arm volumeter.

6.5.2.2   Bioimpedance Assessment

A bioimpedance was introduced because of its ability to assess the amount of extra-cellular fluid. With the currently available bioimpedance devices, it is possible to scan specific body areas and to calculate ratios or L-Dex scores. Despite its ability to assess extracellular fluid, some critical remarks should be made. An edema is mostly fluid in the beginning and becomes progressively fatter in substance due to tissue formation. How well BIA is able to assess these changes needs to be established. Although, L-Dex scores as well as ratios (affected vs unaffected area/limb) are used; different scores and ratios are reported in the literature. Therefore, it is difficult to provide a global recom-mendation on the use of BIA.

Bioimpedance analysis should be used to detect lymphatic transport impairments and diagnose subclinical and early-stage lymphedema in patients at risk for breast can-cer-related lymphedema (stages 0 and 1).[8] (Evidence Quality: Level II reliability, validity and diagnostic accuracy; Recommendation Strength: Grade B):

- an L-Dex score of more than 7.1 should be used as a diagnostic criterion for breast cancer-related lymphedema when no preoperative assessment is available. (Evidence Quality: Level II diagnostic accuracy; Recommendation Strength: Grade B).
- an L-Dex score of more than 10 above preoperative baseline measures should be used as a diagnostic criterion. (Evidence Quality: Level II diagnostic accuracy; Recommendation Strength: Grade B).

In moderate- to late-stage cancer-related lymphedema, as tissue formation occurs BIA may be used as a diagnostic tool; however, clinicians must be aware of the potential for decreasing extracellular fluid even with increased tissue volume.

6.5.2.3 Circumferential Measurements

A circumferential measurement is probably one of the easiest assessments to perform. However, some standardization aspects should be respected:

- First, always use the same type of tape measure. Different tape measures are available with their own specific width.
- Second, be precise in placing the reference marks, use a fine tip pencil or pen.
- Third, different protocols for the assessments of the limbs exist. For clinical practice it is important to train yourself and team in the chosen protocols.
- Fourth, when executing a circumference measurement, always place the tape measure at the same point with respect to the reference point, e.g., always distally or proximally of the reference point.
- Fifth, standardize the pulling pressure; this is mostly done by using the weight of the tape measure. Additionally, instruments like the Perimeter use a fixed weight of 20g at the end of the tape measure.

Circumferential measurement can be used to diagnose upper and lower extremity lymphedema (with or without hand/foot involvement) at stage 1 or greater. (Evidence Quality: Level I reliability, validity and Level II diagnostic accuracy; Recommendation Strength: Grade B).[8]

A volume ratio of 1.04 may be indicative of upper-extremity lymphedema. (Evidence Quality: Level II diagnostic accuracy; Recommendation Strength: Grade B).

Since a calculated volume difference between sides (≥200 mL) is not sensitive enough (as demonstrated by Armer 2005[9]) new cut-off points based on percentages instead of ml are suggested. In the Dutch guidelines, 0-5%, 5-10% and >10% differences are used to define mild, moderate and severe chronic edema, respectively.[1]

If preoperative measures are available, a 5% (in some studies 3% is suggested to diagnose early onset of edema) or greater volume change from baseline above and below the elbow is diagnostic of upper-extremity lymphedema. (Evidence Quality: Level II diagnostic accuracy; Recommendation Strength: Grade B).

Circumferential measurement taken at any single site along the upper extremity, and specifically a difference of 2 cm or more, should not be used as a diagnostic criterion for upper-extremity lymphedema due to poor accuracy. (Evidence Quality: Level II diagnostic accuracy; Recommendation Strength: Grade B).

For **hand or foot lymphedema**, a 'figure-of-eight' method of circumferential measurement may be used as an assessment tool for determining hand/foot volume.[12,13]

For **head and neck lymphedema**, circumferential measurement taken at a single point of the upper neck (under the jawline) may be useful for assessment but has not been studied as a diagnostic test. (Evidence Quality: Level I reliability, Level II validity; no diagnostic accuracy; Recommendation Strength: Expert Opinion)[14]

6.5.2.4   Perometry

Perometry is an opto-electric assessment of the limbs.[11] A limb is scanned every 0.5cm by means of a grid calculating the circumferences. Next, these circumferences are recalculated as a volume by the accompanying software. The volumes of both limbs can be compared and the same diagnostic criteria (e.g., 0-5; 5-10 and >10%) difference apply. Although perometry is very fast in calculating the volumes, its clinical use is impeded by its cost and seldom used in private practices. Therefore, this technique is limited in clinical utility to large centres/hospitals.

6.5.2.5   Tissue Dielectric Constant – MoistureMeter

The MoistureMeter is a device that uses microwaves to assess the amount of water that is present at a defined depth underneath the skin. This device calculates a Tissue Dielectric Constant, or TDC value, and this TDC value is recalculated as a percentage of fluid.[15-19] This device is validated in haemodialysis patients, showing decreasing TDC values as more fluid was evacuated from the body during dialysis. Additionally, reliability values are moderate to excellent. It has been demonstrated that less reliable values (ICC 0.633-0.770) can be obtained from the feet and hands probably due to presence of a dense network of superficial veins. A significantly better reliability is shown for the ankle (ICC >0.970) and lower leg (ICC >0.930), as well as the forearm (ICC >0.900) and biceps (ICC >0.850). TDC values are also reliable for the head and neck region, when assessed at 8 cm below the lower lip.[20]

Important remark

Although several edema assessments have been studied in scientific/clinical studies and showed good clinimetric properties, the possibilities for using edema assessments are defined (read: restricted) by the national health-care system. Belgium's health-care system, for example, only allows hand or foot water displacement techniques for unilateral hand or foot edema. For unilateral edema of the upper or lower limb, Belgium's system has defined its own protocol based on circumference measurements. For all other types of edema, it requests a lympho-scintigraphic investigation. The only exception is made for patients younger than 14 years of age.

More details about these regulations can be found on the website of the RIZIV. A link to this website can be found on the online learning platform Sofia.

A clinical study performed by De Vrieze et al. investigated what would be the best clinical method for assessing arm lymphedema volume.[11] They compared five different assessments (standard water displacement with overflow, inverse volumetry, valgrado water displacement, perimeter circumference and perometer). All assessments had been previously tested (in the original studies) for validity and reliability. Based on the results of this comparative study, the perimeter circumference measurement with calculated volume is the best measurement method for evaluating excessive arm volume over time in terms of reliability, low error rate, low cost, least amount of limitations and the time spent.[11] Also see the protocol of the Perimeter assessment of the arm for a picture of the device.

6.5.2.6 Protocols for the clinical assessment of chronic edema

Water displacement method arm[10]

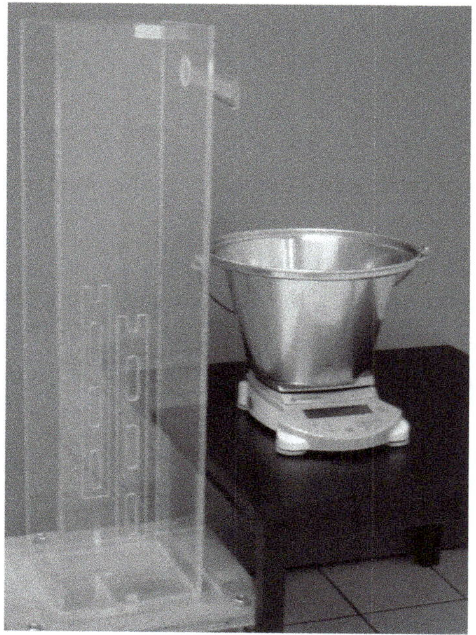

Figure 6.7 Setup of an arm volumeter.

Setup of the volumeter:
- Marking the reference point: mid-humerus = 50% of the distance between the lower edge of the acromium and epicondylus lateralis humeri.
- The patient sits down on a chair next to the volumeter.

- The volumeter is level and filled with water at a temperature of 28 ° C (± 2 ° C).
- The electronic scale, with recipient on it, is set to zero.
- The patient slowly lowers his/her arm into the volumeter until the mark on the arm is level with the mark on the volumeter.
- The water overflows. Wait until the water stops running or until the water drips at a frequency <1 droplet / sec.
- The volume is read on the scale. 1ml = 1gr.
- The procedure is repeated for the other arm.

Water displacement method hand[21]

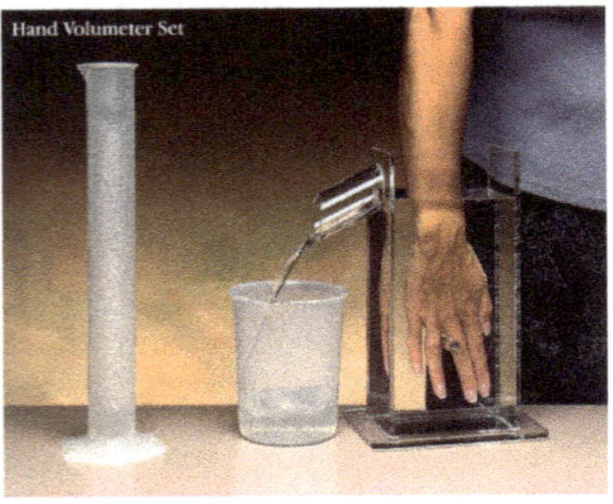

Figure 6.8   Setup of a hand volumeter.

Setup of the hand volumeter:
- The volumeter is placed on a table and is level. It is filled with water at a temperature of 28 ° C (± 2 ° C).
- The electronic scale, with recipient on it, is set to zero.
- The patient slowly lowers his/her hand perpendicularly into the volumeter until the 3rd webspace of the hand reaches the bar in the volumeter.
- The water overflows. Wait until the water stops running or until the water drips at a frequency <1 droplet / sec.
- The volume is read on the scale. 1ml = 1gr.
- The procedure is repeated for the other hand.

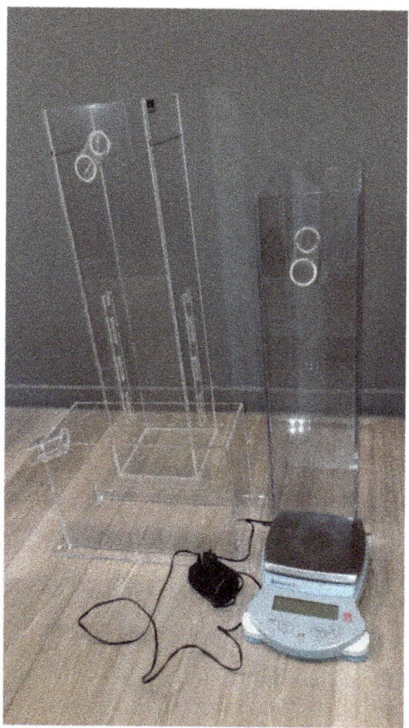

Figure 6.9 Different volumeters, with the foot volumeter in front. To assess a volume, a volumeter is used in combination with an electronic scale.

- The volumeter is placed on the floor and is level. It is filled with water at a temperature of 28 ° C (± 2 ° C).
- The patient sits down on a chair and places both feet next to the volumeter.
- The electronic scale, with recipient on it, is set to zero.
- The patient slowly lowers his/her foot perpendicularly into the volumeter until the foot reaches the bottom of the volumeter.
- The water overflows. Wait until the water stops running or until the water drips at a frequency <1 droplet / sec.
- The volume is read on the scale. 1ml = 1gr.
- The procedure is repeated for the other foot.

Arm perimeter[22]

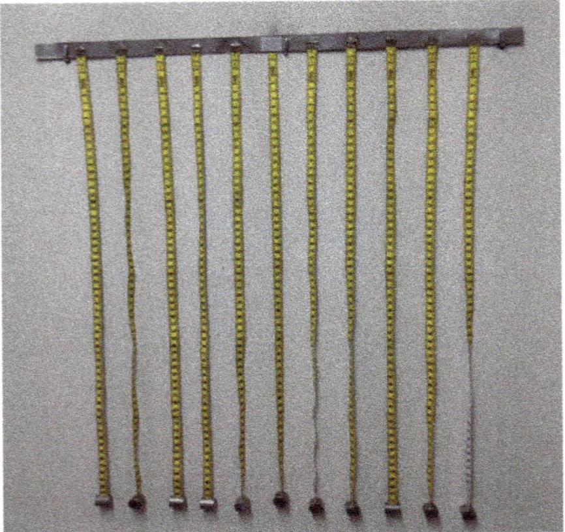

With courtesy of Prof. N. Devoogdt, KU Leuven, UZ Leuven.

Figure 6.10 The perimeter, a flexible rod with 11 tape measures with 4 cm intervals. A weight of 20g is fixed at the end of every tape measure to ensure a standardized pulling force.

- Starting position: seated on a chair, 90° anteflexion of the shoulder with extended elbow and hand supported, for example, on the backrest of a chair.
- Reference point: upper edge olecranon.
- Procedure:
  - Place the lath on the dorsal side of the upper arm (parallel to the upper arm's longitudinal axis) so that the measuring tapes hang down at the lateral side of the arm. (Note: It is possible that, in people with flexion of the elbow, the lath is only parallel to the longitudinal axis of the upper arm and not to the longitudinal axis of the forearm).
  - Place the middle measuring tape around the arm with the proximal edge against the reference point (to determine the circumference at the olecranon).
  - Place the measuring tapes proximal to the olecranon around the arm, first the distal tape measure and then move stepwise proximally (to measure circumferences at 4, 8, 12, 16 and 20cm above the olecranon). Attention: The measuring tapes should always be perpendicular to the longitudinal axis of the arm. Do not tighten the tape measures (the weight at the end of the tape measures provides tension). Make sure that the measuring tapes enclose the arm completely.
  - Read and record arm circumferences. If there is an opening between the lath and the upper arm, press the lath against the upper arm.
  - Remove all measuring tapes, except the middle one.
  - Place the lath on the dorsal side of the forearm (parallel to the longitudinal axis of the forearm).
  - Place the measuring tapes distal to the olecranon around the forearm. Read and record arm circumferences.

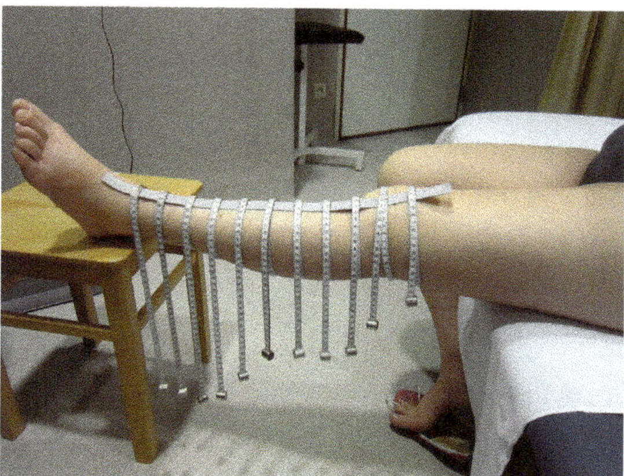

With courtesy of Prof. N. Devoogdt, KU Leuven, UZ Leuven.

Figure 6.11 An example of the use of the perimeter for a lower limb.

- Starting position: Extension of the knee and foot supported (e.g., on a stool). Ask to carry out limited foot flexion, 90° flexion hip.
- Reference point: Upper edge patella.
- Procedure:
  - Place the lath on the dorsal side of the lower leg (parallel to the longitudinal axis of the lower leg) with the distal edge of the first measuring tape against the reference point and with the measuring tapes hanging down at the lateral side of the lower leg.
  - Measure the circumference at the patella and 4, 8, 12, 16, 20, 24, 28, 32, 36 (40) cm below the patella. Place the measuring tapes around the lower leg; place each measuring tape perpendicular to the longitudinal axis of the lower leg. Do not pull the measuring tapes (the weight at the end of the tapes provides tension) Make sure that the measuring tapes enclose the leg completely.
  - Read and record the leg circumferences. If there is space between the leg and the lath, press it against the leg.
  - Remove all measuring tapes. Place the lath on the upper leg (parallel to the longitudinal axis of the upper leg) to measure the circumferences of the upper leg. Make sure the lath doesn't push in the abdomen of the patient.
  - The measuring tape at the patella is placed around the leg with the distal edge at the reference point. Measure the circumferences at 4, 8, 12, 16, 20 (24, 28) cm above the patella. Place all measuring tapes around the upper leg, starting with the measuring tape 4cm above the patella. Place each measuring tape perpendicular to the longitudinal axis of the lower leg. Note the circumferential measurements of the upper leg.

Note:

For practical reasons, it is an option to place the lath on the ventral side of the lower leg against the tibia.

It is often not possible to measure the upper leg using the perimeter, because the measuring tapes are not long enough. In this case, use another method, such as the circumference measurements using a single measuring tape.

Arm circumference measurements

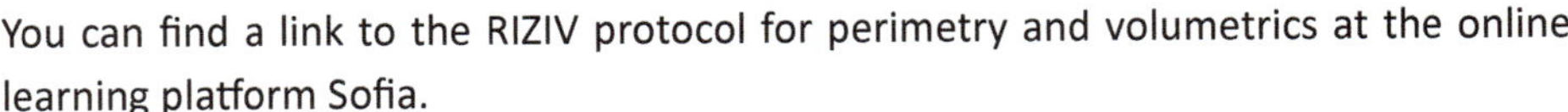

You can find a link to the RIZIV protocol for perimetry and volumetrics at the online learning platform Sofia.

Marking the reference points

Forearm: Place a mark every 4 cm on the line between the top of the os pisiforme and the top of the epicondylus medialis humeri.

Arm: Place a mark every 4 cm on the line between the top of the epicondylus medialis humeri and the deltopectoral groove.

Circumference measurements

The circumference is measured at each mark using a flexible measuring tape; one must ensure that the measuring tape is placed without tension, in the middle of the mark and perpendicularly to the major axis of the segment.

The measurement is done three times and recorded in centimetres and millimetres for each mark. Only the value of the mathematical mean of the three measurements is taken into account for the calculation. The values are rounded upwards in centimetres if they are higher or equal to 0.5. They will be rounded downwards if they are lower than 0.5.

Leg circumference measurements

You can find a link to the RIZIV protocol for perimetry and volumetrics at the online learning platform Sofia.

Marking the reference points

Lower leg: Place a mark every 4 cm on the line between the top of the malleolus lateralis and the end of the fibula.

Upper leg: Place a mark every 4 cm on the line between the top of the condylus lateralis of the femur and the spina iliaca anterior superior.

The circumference is measured at each mark using a flexible measuring tape; one must ensure that the measuring tape is placed without tension, in the middle of the mark and perpendicularly to the major axis of the segment.

The measurement is done three times and recorded in centimetres and millimetres for each mark. Only the value of the mathematical mean of the three measurements is taken into account for the calculation. The values are rounded upwards in centimetres if they are higher or equal to 0.5. They will be rounded downwards if they are lower than 0.5.

Figure 8 of the hand[12]

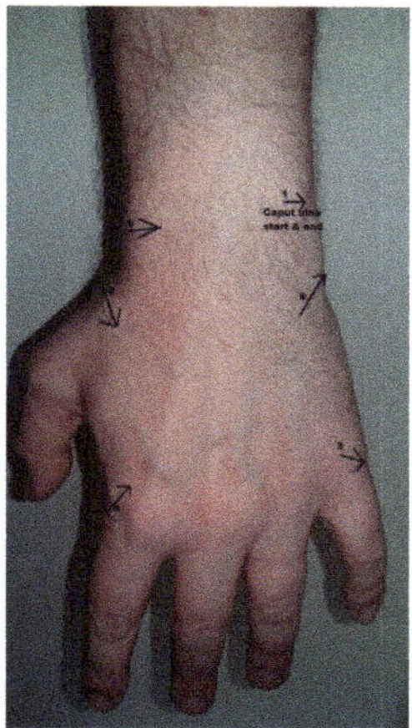

Figure 6.12 Figure 8 of the hand, with arrows denoting the sequence of the application of the tape measure.

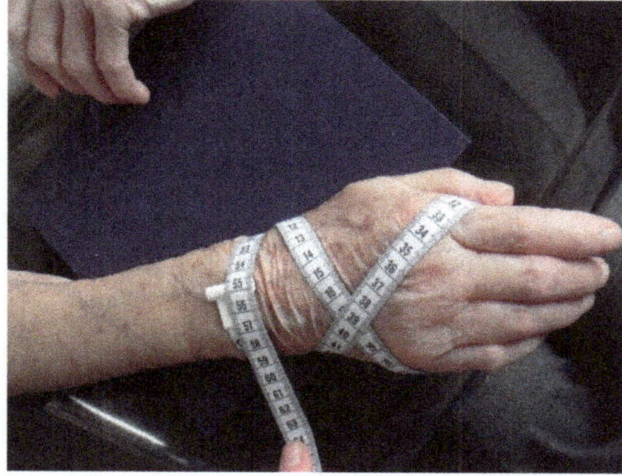

Figure 6.13 Figure 8 method, an example.

The zero mark of the tape measure is placed over the distal aspect of the processus styloideus ulnae, and the tape was drawn across the ventral surface of the wrist to the distal aspect of the processus styloideus radii. Next, the tape measure was drawn diagonally across the dorsum of the hand, brought over the ventral surface of the metacarpophalangeal joints and wrapped diagonally across the dorsum to return to the starting point.

Figure 8 foot[13]

To perform the figure of 8 method, the patient places the ankle in a neutral position. Reference points are put on the distal border of the lateral and medial malleolus and on the proximal border of metatarsal 1 and 5.The tapeline starts at the middle of anterior tibial tendon and the lateral malleolus and goes to the navicular bone proximal of the first metatarsal, crossing the arch of the foot to the base of the fifth metatarsal, towards the distal border of the medial malleolus via the Achilles tendon towards the distal border of the lateral malleolus and ending at the starting point.

Jewelry rings[12]

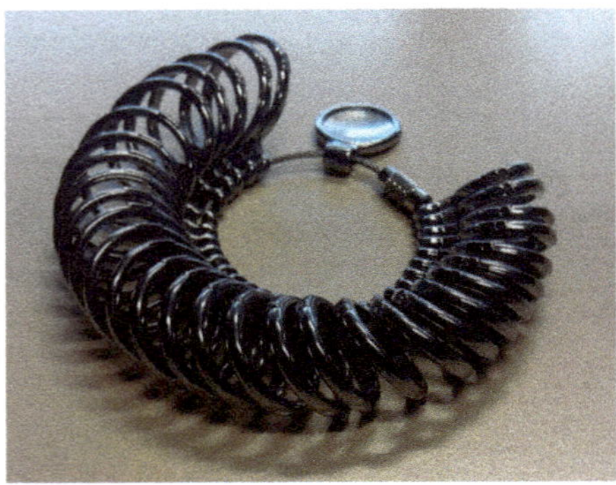
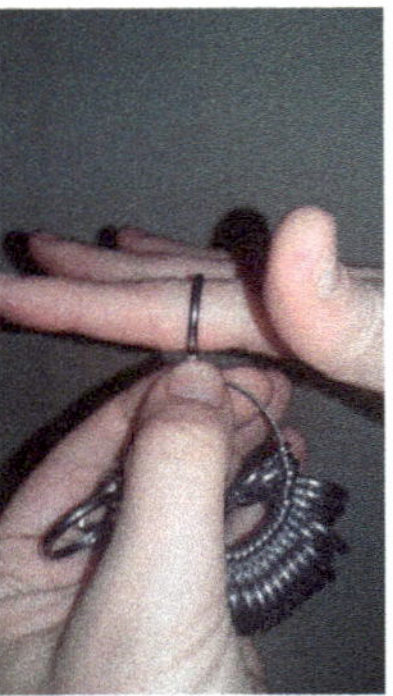

Figure 6.14 The jeweler rings and an example of the execution of the jeweler ring protocol for a middle finger.

For ring and middle finger. Determine the ring that encircles the circumference of the proximal phalanx (widest part) without airspace. Both hands are assessed.

6.6   QUESTIONNAIRES

To cover all health-related quality of lifeissues in patients suffering from chronic edema, it is necessary to look at a biopsychosocial context as well. The International Classification of Functioning, Disability and Health (ICF) is an extensively used framework that describes the health condition of a patient and covers all domains of disability. Functional limitations of the affected limb often have a much greater impact on the quality of life than the increase in the size of a limb. The assessment methods discussed above mainly focus on impairments in functions and structures. For their part, questionnaires can be used to measure activity limitations and participation restrictions. We can make a distinction between generic questionnaires and disease specific questionnaire. The following is an overview of possible questionnaires which can be used for lymphedema patients.

6.6.1 The Norman Questionnaire

The Norman Questionnaire (NQ) was developed in 2001 as a self-reporting questionnaire for the detection of Breast Cancer-Related Lymphedema (BCRL).[23] It contains on questions concerning subjective differences in size of the hands, lower arms and upper arms. In the second part of the NQ, additional questions related to puffiness, feelings of tiredness, tightness of clothing or jewelry, skin indentation, skin texture, pain, hand swelling, writing difficulties, post-exercise swelling and lymphedema in chest, breast or trunk region are scored by the patients themselves. In contrast to the other questionnaires listed below, the NQ aims to detect/diagnose BCRL. In the original study, the clinical use of the NQ was established.[23] A cross-cultural validation of the NQ-Dutch version has been performed, showing a moderate agreement between the NQ-Dutch and clinical assessments for BCRL.[24]

On the online learning platform Sofia, you can find a link to the articles *Reliability and validity of a Dutch Lymphoedema Questionnaire: Cross-cultural validation of the Norman Questionnaire* and *Development and validation of a telephone questionnaire to characterize lymphedema in women treated for breast cancer.*

6.6.2 Lymph-ICF

The Lymph-ICF has a version for the lower limb (Lymph-ICF-LL)[25] and one for the upper limb (Lymph-ICF-UL).[26,27] Both versions contain 28 questions concerning impairments in function, activity limitations and participation restrictions and are designed specifically for lymphedema patients. Five domains are included: physical function, mental function, general tasks/household activities, mobility activities and life domains/social life. The reliability and validity of the Lymph-ICF has been demonstrated for both versions.[25,27]

For a detailed description of these questionnaires, see the article *Lymphoedema Functioning, Disability and Health Questionnaire for Lower Limb Lymphoedema (Lymph-ICF-LL): Reliability and Validity.* You can also read a *Revision of the Lymphedema Functioning, Disability and Health Questionnaire for Upper Limb Lymphedema (Lymph-ICF-UL): Reliability and validity.* A link to these articles is provided on the online learning platform Sofia.

6.6.3 ULL27

The Upper Limb Lymphedema 27 (ULL27) is a self-report questionnaire which consists of 27 questions on a 5-point Likert scale. It measures the effects of lymphedema on health-related quality of life. The questionnaire measures three domains: physical (15 items), psychological (7 items) and social functioning (5 items), with scores ranging from 0 to 100. It is originally a French questionnaire, though a Dutch translation is available. As the name implies, this questionnaire solely applies to lymphedema of the upper limb. Its internal consistency and construct validity has been demonstrated, while its test-retest reliability and content validity has not.[28]

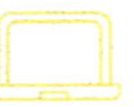

On the online learning platform Sofia, you can find a link to the article *Upper limb lymphedema 27 (ULL27): Dutch translation and validation of an illness-specific-health-related quality of life questionnaire for patients with upper limb lymphedema.*

6.6.4 FLQA-l

The Freiburg Life Quality Assessment (FLQA-l) consists of 92 items and aims to assess the impact of primary and secondary lymphedemain both the lower limb and the upper limb. This valid and reliable questionnaire was developed in German.[29]

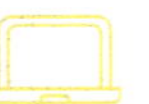

On the online learning platform Sofia, you can find a link to the article *Validation of a short-form of the Freiburg Life Quality Assessment for lymphoedema (FLQA-LS) instrument.*

6.6.5 Generic questionnaires

In addition to the above-mentioned disease-specific questionnaires, several generic questionnaires to assess the daily functioning and quality of life in lymphedema patients can be used as well:

- Disability of the Arm Shoulder and Hand questionnaire (DASH);
- 36-item Short Form Health Survey 36 (SF-36);
- Nottingham Health Profile (NHP);
- Psychosocial Adjustment to Illness Scale (PAIS);
- EORTC;
- Tampa scale for kinesiphobia;
- McGill-QoL.

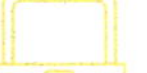

You can find links to all these questionnaires on the online learning platform Sofia.

What the physiotherapist needs to know:

- A comprehensive clinical examination with a focus on the patient interview, inspection and palpation is essential, as functional tests for the lymphatic system are absent.
- A patient interview is essential because it reveals:
    - misbeliefs concerning chronic edema that might hamper treatment;
    - compliance and boundaries issues;
    - unrealistic goal setting by patients.
- Edema assessments focus on the edema volume; however, to grasp the full burden of chronic edema it is important to examine the patient with regard to the ICF model.
- Many edema volume assessments have been found to be valid and reliable, but the national health-care system will define which assessments can be used in clinical practice (focus on reimbursement regulations).

What other health-care workers need to know:

- Physicians can already perform the technical investigation and discuss the results with the patient prior to referral.
- In case of misbeliefs, unrealistic goal setting and low or non-compliance, treatment should also involve counseling by other disciplines (e.g., psychologists) and multidisciplinary meetings should be organized.
- Information from the different questionnaires is valuable to all health-care workers involved in the treatment of patients with chronic edema.

6.7 REFERENCES

1. Damstra RJ, Halk AB. The Dutch lymphedema guidelines based on the International Classification of Functioning, Disability, and Health and the chronic care model. J Vasc Surg Venous Lymphat Disord. 2017;5(5):756-765.
2. The diagnosis and treatment of peripheral lymphedema: 2020 Consensus Document of the International Society of Lymphology. Lymphology. 2020;53(1):3-19.
3. Gebruers N, Verbelen H, De Vrieze T, et al. Current and future perspectives on the evaluation, prevention and conservative management of breast cancer related lymphoedema: A best practice guideline. European journal of obstetrics, gynecology, and reproductive biology. 2017;216:245-253.
4. Thomis S, Dams L, Fourneau I, et al. Correlation Between Clinical Assessment and Lymphofluoroscopy in Patients with Breast Cancer-Related Lymphedema: A Study of Concurrent Validity. Lymphat Res Biol. 2020;18(6):539-548.
5. Pappalardo M, Lin C, Ho OA, Kuo CF, Lin CY, Cheng MH. Staging and clinical correlations of lymphoscintigraphy for unilateral gynecological cancer-related lymphedema. Journal of surgical oncology. 2020;121(3):422-434.

6.   Coleridge-Smith P, Labropoulos N, Partsch H, Myers K, Nicolaides A, Cavezzi A. Duplex ultrasound investigation of the veins in chronic venous disease of the lower limbs--UIP consensus document. Part I. Basic principles. Eur J Vasc Endovasc Surg. 2006;31(1):83-92.

7.   De Vrieze T, Vos L, Gebruers N, et al. Protocol of a randomised controlled trial regarding the effectiveness of fluoroscopy-guided manual lymph drainage for the treatment of breast cancer-related lymphoedema (EFforT-BCRL trial). European journal of obstetrics, gynecology, and reproductive biology. 2018;221:177-188.

8.   Levenhagen K, Davies C, Perdomo M, Ryans K, Gilchrist L. Diagnosis of Upper-Quadrant Lymphedema Secondary to Cancer: Clinical Practice Guideline From the Oncology Section of APTA. Rehabil Oncol. 2017;35(3):E1-e18.

9.   Armer JM, Stewart BR. A comparison of four diagnostic criteria for lymphedema in a post-breast cancer population. Lymphat Res Biol. 2005;3(4):208-217.

10.   Gebruers N, Truijen S, Engelborghs S, De Deyn PP. Volumetric evaluation of upper extremities in 250 healthy persons. Clin Physiol Funct Imaging. 2007;27(1):17-22.

11.   De Vrieze T, Gebruers N, Tjalma WA, et al. What is the best method to determine excessive arm volume in patients with breast cancer-related lymphoedema in clinical practice? Reliability, time efficiency and clinical feasibility of five different methods. Clinical rehabilitation. 2019;33(7):1221-1232.

12.   Gebruers N, Van Soom T, Verbelen H, De Vrieze T. Reliability of Jeweler Rings and a Revised Figure-of-Eight Circumference Protocol for the Assessment of Finger and Hand Circumferences. Lymphat Res Biol. 2021.

13.   Devoogdt N, Cavaggion C, Van der Gucht E, et al. Reliability, Validity, and Feasibility of Water Displacement Method, Figure-of-Eight Method, and Circumference Measurements in Determination of Ankle and Foot Edema. Lymphat Res Biol. 2019;17(5):531-536.

14.   Balci FL, DeGore L, Soran A. Breast Cancer--Related Lymphedema in Elderly Patients. Topics in Geriatric Rehabilitation. 2012;28(4):243-253.

15.   Birkballe S, Jensen MR, Noerregaard S, Gottrup F, Karlsmark T. Can tissue dielectric constant measurement aid in differentiating lymphoedema from lipoedema in women with swollen legs? Br J Dermatol. 2014;170(1):96-102.

16.   Jensen MR, Birkballe S, Nørregaard S, Karlsmark T. Validity and interobserver agreement of lower extremity local tissue water measurements in healthy women using tissue dielectric constant. Clin Physiol Funct Imaging. 2012;32(4):317-322.

17.   Mayrovitz HN. Assessing Upper and Lower Extremities Via Tissue Dielectric Constant: Suitability of Single Versus Multiple Measurements Averaged. Lymphat Res Biol. 2019;17(3):316-321.

18.   Mayrovitz HN, Lorenzo-Valido C, Pieper E, Thomas A. Forearm and biceps circumferential variations in skin tissue dielectric constant and firmness. Lymphology. 2020;53(4):204-211.

19.   Mayrovitz HN, Weingrad DN, Brlit F, Lopez LB, Desfor R. Tissue dielectric constant (TDC) as an index of localized arm skin water: differences between measuring probes and genders. Lymphology. 2015;48(1):15-23.

20.   Purcell A, Nixon J, Fleming J, McCann A, Porceddu S. Measuring head and neck lymphedema: The «ALOHA» trial. Head Neck. 2016;38(1):79-84.

21.   King TI, 2nd. The effect of water temperature on hand volume during volumetric measurement using the water displacement method. J Hand Ther. 1993;6(3):202-204.

22.   Devoogdt N, Lemkens H, Geraerts I, et al. A new device to measure upper limb circumferences: validity and reliability. International angiology: a journal of the International Union of Angiology. 2010;29(5):401-407.

23.   Norman SA, Miller LT, Erikson HB, Norman MF, McCorkle R. Development and validation of a telephone questionnaire to characterize lymphedema in women treated for breast cancer. Physical therapy. 2001;81(6):1192-1205.

24.   De Groef A, De Vrieze T, Dams L, et al. Reliability and validity of a Dutch Lymphoedema Questionnaire: Cross-cultural validation of the Norman Questionnaire. European journal of cancer care. 2020;29(4):e13242.

25.   Devoogdt N, De Groef A, Hendrickx A, et al. Lymphoedema Functioning, Disability and Health Questionnaire for Lower Limb Lymphoedema (Lymph-ICF-LL): reliability and validity. Physical therapy. 2014;94(5):705-721.

26. De Vrieze T, Gebruers N, Nevelsteen I, et al. Responsiveness of the Lymphedema Functioning, Disability, and Health Questionnaire for Upper Limb Lymphedema in Patients with Breast Cancer-Related Lymphedema. Lymphat Res Biol. 2020;18(4):365-373.

27. De Vrieze T, Vos L, Gebruers N, et al. Revision of the Lymphedema Functioning, Disability and Health Questionnaire for Upper Limb Lymphedema (Lymph-ICF-UL): Reliability and Validity. Lymphat Res Biol. 2019;17(3):347-355.

28. Viehoff PB, van Genderen FR, Wittink H. Upper limb lymphedema 27 (ULL27): Dutch translation and validation of an illness-specific health-related quality of life questionnaire for patients with upper limb lymphedema. Lymphology. 2008;41(3):131-138.

29. Augustin M, Bross F, Földi E, Vanscheidt W, Zschocke I. Development, validation and clinical use of the FLQA-I, a disease-specific quality of life questionnaire for patients with lymphedema. Vasa. 2005;34(1):31-35.

7 TREATMENT OF PATIENTS WITH CHRONIC EDEMA

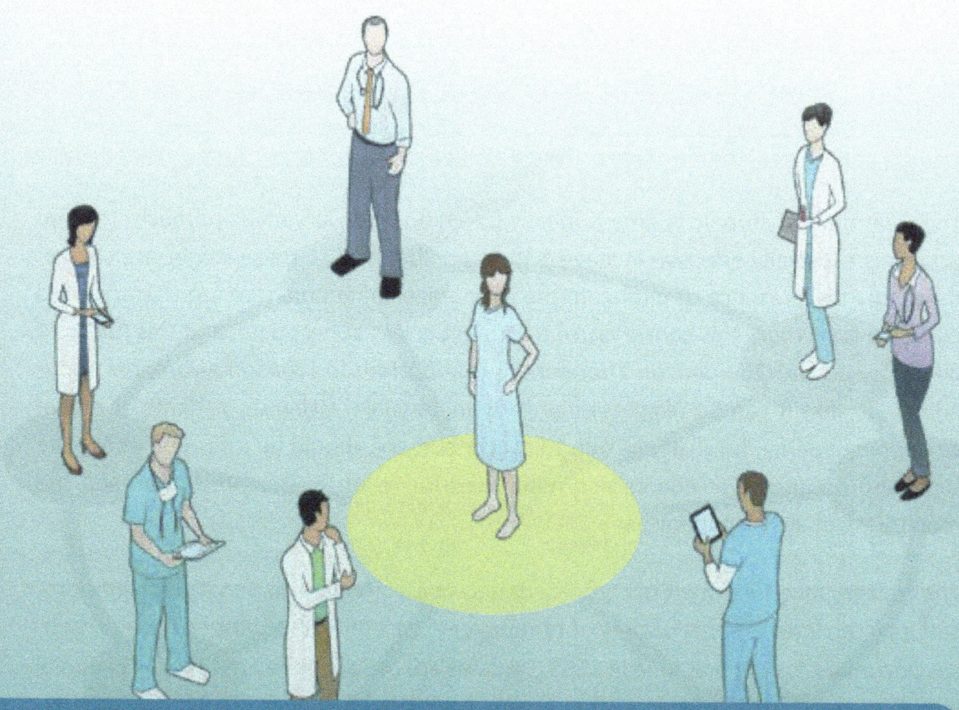

The learning objectives for this chapter are:

- Knowledge of the conservative treatment of chronic edema
- Provide background knowledge on the consensus treatment and its different pillars
- Provide scientific evidence on the different pillars of the consensus treatment to improve decision making processes for patients with chronic edema

7.1   INTRODUCTION

Different guidelines are available for the treatment of chronic edema.[1-4] Based on these guidelines and original research we will discuss the currently accepted treatment for chronic edema. We will focus on the conservative treatment of chronic edema. Although several surgical procedures such as lympho-lymphatic anastomosis, lympho-venous anastomosis, lymph node transplantation and debulking techniques like the lipolymphosuction are available, they will not be discussed in this book. If a patient has questions concerning surgery, it is best to refer them to surgeons specialized into these kind of procedures for further information.

7.2   CONSERVATIVE TREATMENT OF CHRONIC EDEMA

The treatment of chronic edema is mostly based on a conservative approach. This approach is especially effective in stage 1 to stage 2b, because these stages are characterized by the presence of pitting. In the later stages of edema that are characterized by tissue formation, this conservative treatment is less appropriate, and this needs to be discussed with the patient. Therefore, it is important to broaden awareness about edema so that it can be diagnosed as early as possible. Likewise, patients at risk of developing edema, for instance due to cancer surgery, should be informed about the signs and symptoms of edema and monitored for its onset (for prevention and the monitoring of at-risk patients, see Chapter 5).

The conservative treatment of chronic edema is based on international guidelines provided by the International Society of Lymphology (ISL). The ISL published their consensus document for the first time in 1995. Updates are usually done after the ISL biannual world congress, with the most recent update having been done in 2019.[1,5] The International Lymphedema Framework also provides best-practice guidelines.

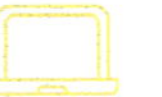 You can find a link to the freely consultable guidelines of the International Lymphedema Framework on the online learning platform Sofia.

The conservative treatment of chronic edema is referred to as the Complex Decongestive Therapy or Complex Physical Therapy, CDT or CPT respectively, and divided into two distinct phases.

- The first phase is called the **intensive treatment phase** or **reduction phase**. The main goal of the intensive treatment is to reduce the edema volume significantly.
- The second phase is called the **maintenance phase**. The main goal is to maintain the edema reduction. The maintenance phase is often life-long. It is therefore very important that patient receives correct and extensive information about their treatment and the responsibilities that go with it.

> **Remark**
>
> Although the aim of conservative treatment is edema volume reduction and its maintenance, it is also important to discuss the broader picture with regard to the ICF-model. It is important to understand the request of help from a patient with regard to the activities in daily life and their participation requests (work and leisure time related). To give one example: many patients are reluctant to wear the compression garments at certain events (social events, holidays but also in the workplace). It is therefore important to discuss the possibilities of night-time management (wearing the garments while sleeping) to better maintain the compression, as otherwise some patients would might choose not to wear their compression garments.

The main pillars of therapeutic modalities of the CDT are:[1]

- skin care;
- manual lymphatic drainage (MLD);
- compression therapy (bandaging during the intensive phase and compression garments during the maintenance phase);
- exercise therapy (both aerobic as well as resistance training).

In addition to the main four pillars, different other modalities can be added to the conservative treatment. For instance, if a patient suffers from obesity or being overweight, a diet needs to be installed in **collaboration with a dietician**. A diet also needs to be discussed with patients who have protein-losing enteropathies or low albumin levels. For patients who have difficulty accepting the diagnosis or the chronicity of the problem, psychological support needs be added to the conservative treatment in **collaboration with a psychologist**. If patients are suffering from severe (open) wounds, wound care needs to be established in **collaboration with a wound nurse**.

Other therapeutic modalities as well as technical investigations are described in the consensus document as well.[1] (For the technical investigations, see Chapter 6).

Complex Physical Therapy or Complex Decongestive Therapy (CPT/CDT)[1]

Phase 1: Intensive treatment (decongestion)	Phase 2: Maintenance (self-management)
Duration: ~2-4 weeks; however, shorter periods of decongestion have been demonstrated	Duration: undefined in time; often life-long; self-management, responsibility of the patient
Aim: volume reduction	Aim: volume maintenance (no further reduction)
Methods (modalities are combined): • **skin care;** • **manual lymphatic drainage;** • **compression bandaging (short stretch, high stiffness);** • **exercises.**	Methods: self-management (often): • skin care; • self-MLD or no MLD; • compression garments (flat knit); • exercises.

Table 7.1   Schematic overview of the main pillars described in the ISL consensus document.

Concerning CDT/CPT, there is sufficient evidence supporting its efficacy in reducing and maintaining the edema volume. However, due to the combination of the different pillars into one treatment session, CDT is time consuming. In many countries the treatment time is limited by reimbursement policies. It is therefore important to use the therapy as effectively as possible and reassess the importance of the different pillars of the consensus document. In the following sections the importance of each individual pillar will be discussed.

7.2.1   Skin care

Skin care comprises some essential recommendations for patients with chronic edema that aim to limit as much as possible an exacerbation of the edema due to an aggravation of the skin condition. It is most important to avoid all kind of wounds, even the very little ones like insect bites, because every skin defect poses the potential risk of an inflammatory process or infection. In addition to wound prevention, keeping the skin well-nourished is a very important part of skin care. Well-nourished skin is more elastic and more capable of enduring the compression provided by bandages or garments and is less vulnerable to wounds or infection. Several (specific) lotions are available for nourshing and moisturizing the skin. Sometimes different lotions need to be tested by the patient to find the most appropriate one. Low-pH and perfume-free soaps and body lotions are recommended. Although most of the recommendations regarding skin care are very obvious, it is necessary to discuss these recommendations with the patient. Again, the patient is responsible for the meticulous skin care and should be informed accordingly.

Since meticulous skin care is of the utmost importance for patients suffering from edema and the patients themselves and their network are responsible for the skin care, we will list the concerns along with the appropriate actions and timing. The instructions in table 7.2 are for patients with an intact skin[6-9] (for patients with severe wounds, collaboration with a wound nurse and dermatologist is called for and tailored skin care needs to be discussed with the patients and the team providing treatment).[10]

Concern	Negative effect	Action and timing
Heat	Increased net filtration by vasodilatation	• Avoid/stay away from heat sources like sunbathing, taking a hot bath, sauna, steam bath. • Take a shower instead of a bath
Moisturizing of the skin	Skin becomes very dry due to the edema as well as the wearing of compression garments; dry skin becomes flaky and is more easily damaged and /or irritated	• Use a moisturizing cream, preferably in the evening after showering. In this way the cream can nourish the skin during sleep • Use a sufficient amount of cream (most patients use far to little cream, one fingertip of cream should be used for the surface of the palm of your hand)
Minor wounds (scratches, insect bites, cuts, skin indurations)	Minor skin breaks can cause serious skin infections or erysipelas	• Disinfect the wound immediately, even insect bites • Be very careful with manicures/pedicures (have them done by a medical professional) • Always have some disinfectant with you when you go out • Dry the skin entirely (especially between the toes) to avoid fissures
Weight	Increased weight results in increased tissue and will increase net filtration, increasing the lymphatic load	• Maintain a normal body weight as much as possible • In case of overweight or obesity → reduce weight (collaborate with a dietician) • Normal weight means avoiding an increase in body weight
Protect yourself	Performing ADL tasks can provoke injury/wounds	Wear protective clothing when gardening or performing tasks with the risk of injury
Avoid restrictive clothing	Lymph flow can be hampered in areas with restrictive clothing	Be careful with wearing belts, shoes, small bra straps, ...
Blood samples and blood pressure measurement	Exacerbation of the edema due to tourniquet and small infection from needle punctures (though the risk is low)	Avoid having blood samples and blood pressure taken on the edematous limb

Table 7.2 Skin care instructions for patients with an intact skin.

As mentioned, the recommendations in table 7.2 are obvious. However, different health-care workers have the opportunity to inform patients of them. Recommendations are not always the same between health-care workers, which can confuse the patient and this should be avoided at all times.[11] Therefore, it is important to discuss the recommendation as a team (all health-care workers that advise this patient) and provide consistent information to a patient. Also, there is a difference between the knowledge of these recommendations among patients at risk for chronic edema due to other aetiologies compared to BCRL patients in that the latter are more aware of the recommendations.[11] It is thus very important to repeat the recommendations to all patients at risk for chronic edema. Different health-care workers should make the same recommendations; this can best be achieved by a multidisciplinary approach and providing a joint brochure or leaflet containing the recommendations.

7.2.2   Manual lymphatic drainage (MLD)

In recent years nothing has been the subject of more debate at the international level than the use of manual lymphatic drainage (MLD). In 1892 Alexander von Winiwarter described his MLD techniques for the treatment of lymphedema. Next, in the 1930s, a Danish biologist by the name of Emil Vodder became interested in treating diseases related to the lymphatic system. He demonstrated his MLD techniques at the health congress (foire de santé) in Paris in 1936. MLD ad modum Vodder is used worldwide, although several other schools of MLD exist. Some examples are Casley-Smith, Lehrner, Leduc and Földi. It is thus important to realize that 'MLD' can involve different maneuvers depending on the school, with pressures varying as well as the sequence.

Something that all schools of MLD have in common is that the therapy is based on a normal anatomy of the lymphatic system. In other words, the techniques were developed for a normal anatomy and physiology of the lymphatic system. This is called the blind application of MLD.

With respect to the blind application of MLD for treating chronic edema, several strong primary studies[12-14] as well as strong systematic review[15,16] and meta-analytic[17] data are available, with most of the results being obtained from a sample of BCRL patients. All of these studies concluded that MLD has only a limited effect (only 7% of total edema volume reduction) or no effect at all. This evidence calls for a critical mind when it comes to the blind application of MLD.

Another issue that warrants critical appraisal is the use of MLD as a preventative treatment for reducing the risk of chronic edema. This topic has been especially investigated with respect to BCRL and these studies have shown that MLD cannot prevent BCRL.[15,18,19] Therefore, there is no scientific grounds for prescribing MLD only after surgical procedures that involve the resection of lymph tissue and lymph nodes. By contrast, the prescription of physical therapy can be very useful for postoperative rehabilitation encompassing exercises for mobility, strength and endurance with a focus on functioning.[20] The prevention of chronic edema is thoroughly discussed in Chapter 5.

Based on the evidence, the conclusion regarding the blind application of MLD should be that MLD has no or only a clinically limited contribution to the reduction of edema volumes. This is an important finding, since MLD is a time-consuming part of the CDT. The blind application of MLD assumes that the lymphatic anatomy of the patient is normal. However, the anatomy of the lymphatic system changes significantly due to surgery and/or radiation therapy. Even in primary lymphedema, an altered anatomy can be expected. Evidence on the effectiveness of MLD after the lymphatic anatomy has been visualized is still lacking.

To provide this last piece of the puzzle a three-armed RCT was conducted to investigate the effectiveness of lymphofluoroscopy-guided MLD. This RCT was called the EFforT-BCRL trial and was conducted as a multi-centre RCT in Belgium.[21] A total of five hospitals participated in the recruitment and treatment of patients. Patients suffering from BCRL who were referred for intensive decongestive therapy were randomized into one of three groups. The recruited patients received three weeks of intensive CDT. At the end of the intensive treatment phase, the patients received a custom-made compression sleeve and glove (flat-knit technology, compression class 2 or 3). Next, the patients were followed for an additional year. The only difference in the treatment of the three groups was the application of the MLD. In one group, traditional blind MLD (based on the common schools of MLD) was performed in addition to the other pillars of CDT. The second group received the experimental lymphofluoroscopy-guided MLD (based on the Fill & Flush techniques[22]) in addition to CDT. The third group received a placebo therapy by adding a sham MLD to CDT. All three groups were alike for all baseline variables and stages of BCRL.

The results of the EFforT-BCRL trial[21] confirm that the contribution of MLD is nonexistent in a sample of patients with BCRL. A significant, yet equal reduction of edema volumes was achieved among all three groups (including a placebo group). No significant differences were found between the three groups at any point in time. These results confirm that MLD is not the most important treatment modality of CDT. The emphasis should be on the combination of skin care, compression and exercise. The use of MLD in CDT for the treatment of BCRL can no longer be motivated based on scientific evidence for the treatment of BCRL.

7.2.3　Compression therapy

The aim of the compression therapy in the complex decongestive therapy is different among the two phases of CDT. Also, the materials used will differ between the two phases since the goals are set differently.

During the **first phase** of CDT, reducing the edema volume is the essential aim. As such, we will need to use compression systems that can be easily adjusted to the changing edema volume during the different treatment sessions. In practice, this means using short stretch (multilayer) bandages and Velcro or compression systems.

During the **second phase**, the aim is to maintain the edema reduction as much as possible. In other words, it is important that compression systems resist edema formation or recurrence of the edema volume. This goal is most often achieved by implementing compression garments (e.g., sleeves, stockings, panties, gloves). Bandaging during the maintenance phase can still be done with an equal result as compared to compression.[23,24] However, bandaging is more time-consuming and cumbersome and many patients will choose compression garments.

7.2.3.1　Basic principles and laws used in bandaging

These basic principles apply to all bandaging materials used in both phases of CDT.[25]

First, a choice needs to be made depending of the level of activity performed by the patient. As depicted in figure 7.1, two main situations occur: either the patient is sedentary (e.g., wheelchair bound or bedridden or highly inactive, lacking motivation) or the patient can perform at least some physical activities and is motivated to do so.

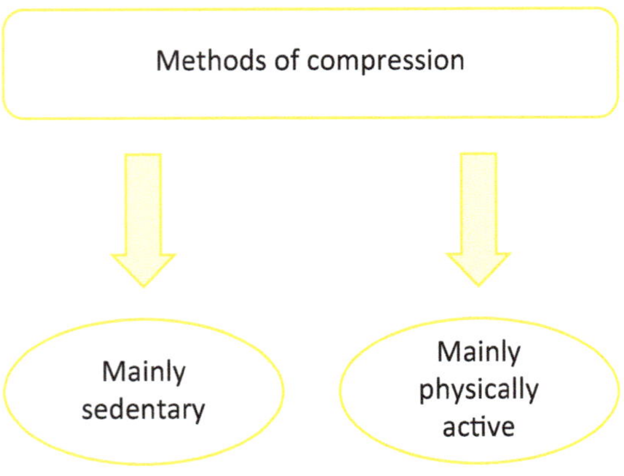

Figure 7.1　Two main situations, depending on the patient's level of activity.

Next, we need to determine which type of compression or support is most beneficial to the patient. Additionally, we need to determine the magnitude of the compression system as well as the sub-bandage pressure with regard to the type of patient.[25] In table 7.3 one can see the difference in application of compression materials.

	Compression	
Type of compression	High elasticity	Non-elastic/short stretch
Resting pressure	Very high pressures at rest (low comfort at night)	Low to moderate pressures at rest (comfort at night)
Working pressure	High pressure yet low alterations in pressure during muscle contractions (muscle pump activation)	High pressure and high fluctuations in pressure during muscle pump activation
Single layer	Delivers constant (low) pressure	Delivers constant (low) pressure
Multilayer	Delivers graded (high) pressure	Delivers graded (high) pressure
Type of patient	Sedentary/ bedridden/ low compliance	Normal activity level/ compliant to exercise
Condition	Venous problems/ open wounds and chronic edema in low compliant patients	Chronic edema, especially after loading conditions

Table 7.3 Difference in the application of compression materials.

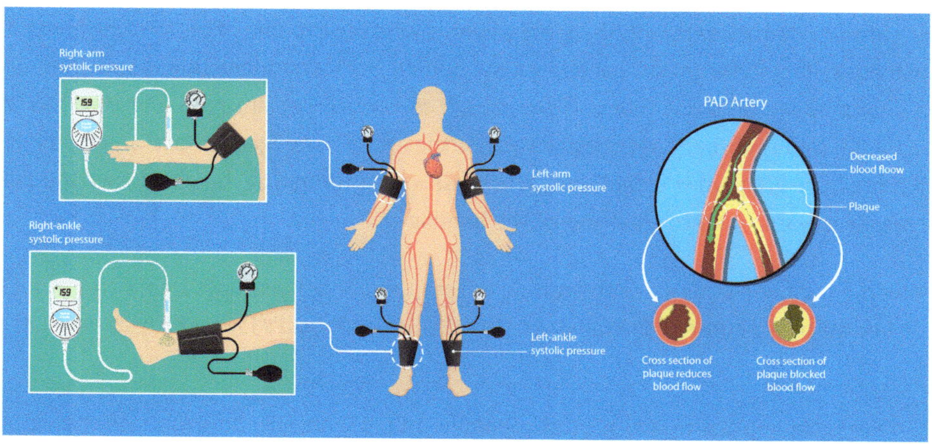

Figure 7.2 Ankle Brachial Index (ABI).

As a therapist/caregiver treating patients with chronic edema, Ankle Brachial Index (ABI) must always be taken into account. Therefore, it is important that you perform the ABI investigation (figure 7.2) or have the investigation done by the referring physician. The results of the ABI will limit the choices you can make as a therapist with respect to applying bandages.

In a healthy patient the ABI is equal to 1. When the ABI is lower than 1, there is a suspicion of a peripheral arterial disease (PAD). PAD is characterized by a reduction of the lumen (mostly due to atherosclerotic changes) of the arteries. As a result, these arteries can be fully compressed more easily, resulting in a blocked arterial flow (= critical ischaemia). Depending on the severity of the PAD, restrictions apply to the use of compression bandages. Between 0.8 and 1 we can continue with all types of compression, although it is preferable to use multicomponent bandages because of the lower resting pressure. A lower resting pressure will compress the lumen of an artery less in comparison with a high resting pressure. For ABIs between 0.5 and 0.8, we will use multicomponent bandages with a low to moderate sub-bandage pressure. If an ABI of <0.5 (critical ischaemia) is measured, it is no longer possible to provide compression bandaging.[25] When the ABI <0.5, the risk of a full compression of the lumen becomes too high. Although a normal ABI = 1, an ABI of higher than 1 is a possibility. In patients with arteriosclerosis, or hardening of the arterial wall, and in patients with diabetes, the ABI will be higher than 1. Arteriosclerosis can mimic PAD. Therefore, in patients with suspected arteriosclerosis, an ABI of 1.3 or higher correlated well with PAD; however, additional investigation (e.g., angiography) may be necessary to establish the safety of the application of compression bandaging. In these cases, referral to a physician is mandatory.

In chronic edema treatment, there are patients who are capable of performing physical activities. Patients with chronic edema will benefit from a bandage that is stiff, that has a sub-bandage pressure that is high enough to control net filtration and that has at least the same sub-bandage pressure across the entire bandaged surface or a gradient. If a pressure gradient is established, the pressure is maximal at the distal part and decreases towards the proximal end of the bandage.[4]

When bandaging patients with chronic edema, two important laws apply and should be known by executer of the bandage. The first law is **Pascal's law**, which states that:

> "Pressure applied to any part of a confined fluid transmits to every other part with no loss. The pressure acts with equal force on all equal areas of the confining walls and perpendicular to the walls."

This is the basic principle of any hydraulic system. Therefore, in chronic edema it is important to create this confined container by applying a stiff (limited elasticity) bandage.

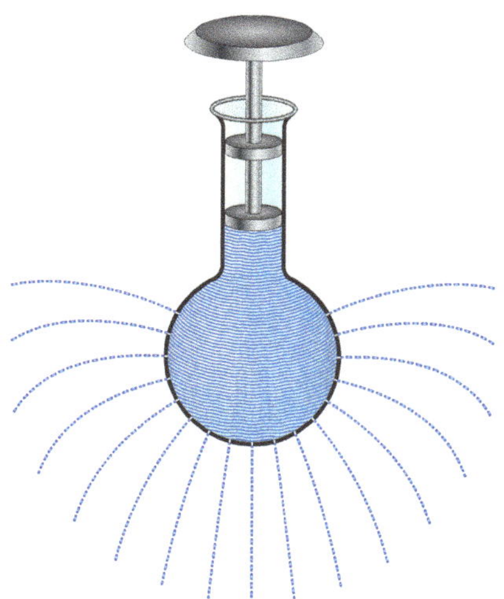

A representation of the effects of Pascal's law in a confined container. In the treatment of patients with chronic edema, we establish the confined container by applying a stiff bandage.

The second law is **Laplace's law**, which states that the sub-bandage pressure is influenced by the amount of tension used by the therapist, the number of layers applied to the skin, the circumference of the limb and bandage width. The law can be written as:

$$\text{subbandage pressure} = \frac{(\text{tension})\,(\#\text{ of layers})\,(\text{constant})}{(\text{circumference of limb})\,(\text{bandage width})}$$

Looking at Laplace's formula, it is clear that sub-bandage pressure will increase if higher tension is applied or more layers are used. Vice versa, a lower sub-bandage pressures is achieved on increased circumferences and when wider bandages are used. During the application of a compression system, a therapist should always keep these laws in mind in order to create the best compression system for any patient.

Laplace's law is also important when looking at the geometry of the bandaged surface, especially different radiuses that can be present on the same part of the body. Parts of the body with a smaller radius will experience higher sub-bandage pressures. Take this information into account when applying padding. Padding will make it possible to increase the radius and help to decrease high pressure points. The effect of different radiuses is clearly demonstrated in figure 7.4.

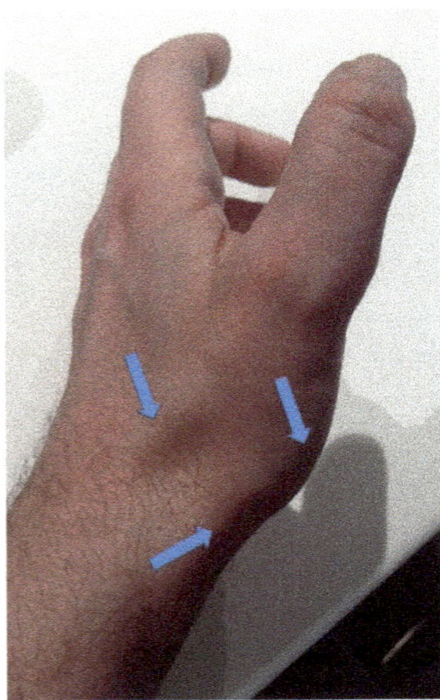

Arrows define the areas with small radiuses at the wrist, and the possible risk of pressure points that can experienced as uncomfortable by the patient.

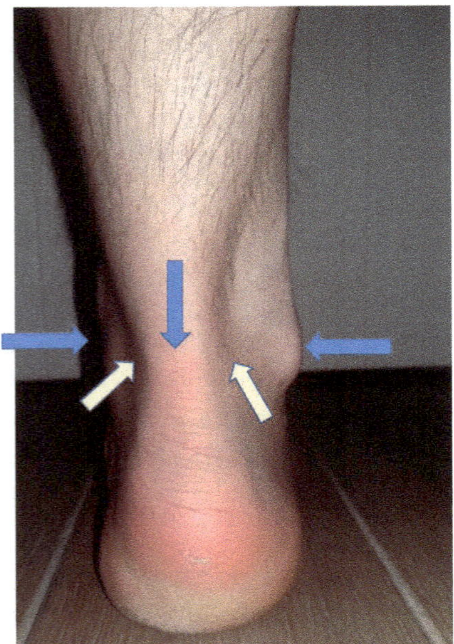

Blue arrows define the areas with small radiuses at the ankle, and the possible risk of pressure points that can experienced as uncomfortable by the patient. White arrows depict the areas with limited to no pressure if no padding is added to the bandage.

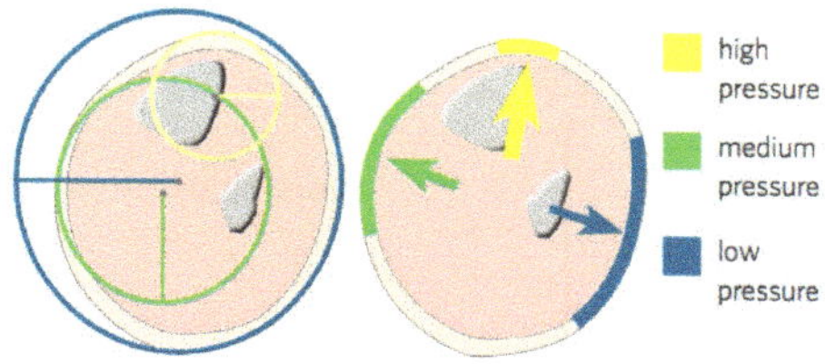

Figure 7.6 Geometry and sub-bandage pressure. Small radiuses have a high sub-bandage pressure and vice versa. Cross sections through the lower right leg showing how different pressures may be generated according to the radius of curvature of the leg.

If we are confronted with different radiuses, we need to apply padding material to smoothen the radiuses and to avoid pressure points. Pressure points are experienced by the patients as annoying and even painful areas underneath the bandage. Sometimes these pressure points are the reason that patients take off their bandage. If this happens the treatment effect of the bandage is lost, thereby extending the intensive treatment phase. The opposite can also exist, meaning that after the application of a bandage, we have areas with very low sub-bandage pressure (e.g., the cavity between the Achilles tendon and the malleoli). If this happens, these areas will fill with the edema fluid, reducing the treatment effect. Again, padding will help to overcome this problem. By filling the cavity with padding material we will be able to increase the sub-bandage pressure.

When applying a compression bandage or system, working pressure and resting pressure are important principles to understand. Working pressure is defined as the alterations in sub-bandage pressure during activity (muscle pump). Resting pressure is the sub-bandage pressure experienced in a resting state with the bandage in place. In addition to the working and resting pressure, bandages are also defined by two indexes: the Static Stiffness Index (SSI) and the Dynamic Stiffness Index (DSI). Static stiffness can be defined as the change in sub-bandage pressure when a patient changes from a supine position (low sub-bandage pressure) to an upright standing position (higher sub-bandage pressure).[26-28] The higher the SSI, the stiffer the bandage is applied to the limb. Dynamic stiffness can be defined as the difference between the minimum and maximum sub-bandage pressure during activity (muscle pump).[29] Again, the higher the DSI, the stiffer the bandage is applied. For the treatment of chronic edema, a high DSI will be more effective in supporting lymphatic flow. Figure 7.7 demonstrates the effect of different types of bandaging on working pressure and resting pressure. SSI is also demonstrated.

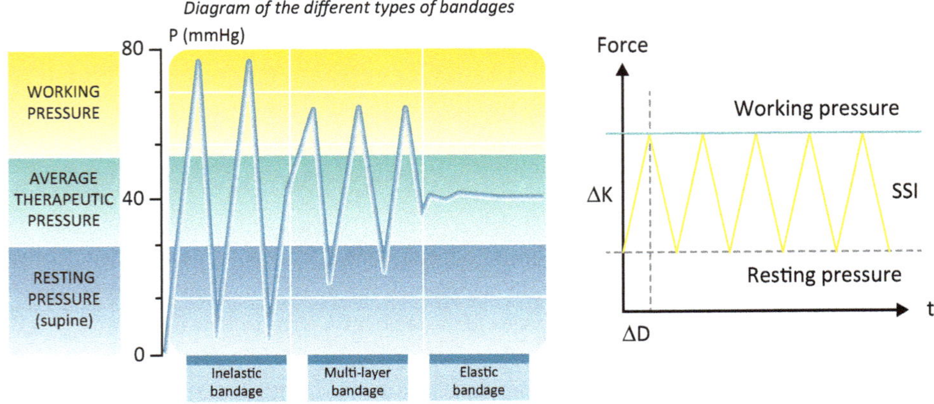

Figure 7.7 Relationship between the type of material used for a bandage and the sub-bandage pressure.

7.2.3.2 Compression therapy during phase 1 of CDT

During the first phase of CDT (aim = edema volume reduction), different types of bandages or compression systems can be used. During this phase (limited to a maximum of 4-6 weeks), it is important that the compression bandage/system is adjustable to the decreasing edema volume. The application of short stretch bandages is most common, and is often considered to be the gold standard. Short stretch (max 30% of elasticity) bandages are cheap and recyclable and are applied as a multilayer bandages or part of a multicomponent bandage. Short stretch bandages need to be reapplied daily (by a physical therapist/spouse/nurse) because the sub-bandage will decrease significantly overnight. Actually, the sub-bandage pressure of short stretch bandages will be decreased by 20-50% over a period of 2 hours. In an ideal situation, short stretch bandages would be re-applied every 2 to 4 hours.[30]

Next, an example of an individual pressure curve of a healthy subject is shown, including 1 hour of mountainbiking between 1H and 2H. 14H is an assessment that takes place after a night's rest.

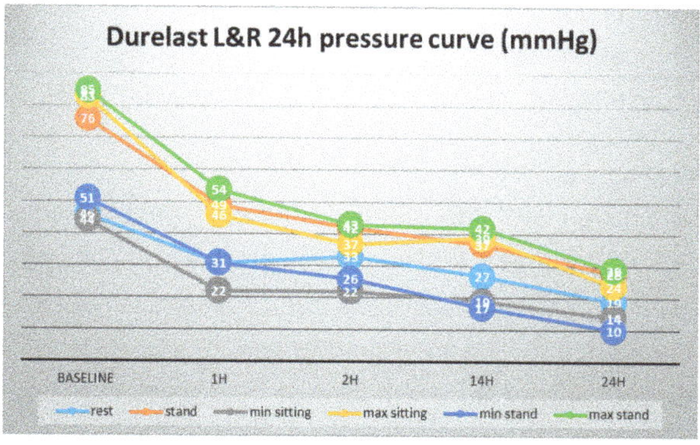

Figure 7.8 A pressure curve of 24 hours for a short stretch bandage. The graph shows a decrease in sub-bandage pressure of nearly 50% after 2h and approximately 75% after 24h.

Keeping in mind that the sub-bandage pressure will drop significantly and that re-applying the bandage is mostly impossible, it is important to aim for a sufficient high application pressure of the bandage. Of course, whenever possible, a short stretch bandage that can be re-applied multiple times (every 2-4 hours) during one day (by the patient or a relative) will be much more effective and speed up the reduction in edema volume. Partsch et al. have investigated the best target pressures that should be achieved after application of a short stretch bandage.[31] It is important to train yourself in the correct application of bandages. Most often the pressure will be too high on the upper limb and too low on the lower limb. The target pressures are different for the upper limb (30-50 mmHg) and lower limb (50-70 mmHg). These target pressures should be assessed directly after application with the patient in a supine position.

The different parts of a short stretch multicomponent or multilayer bandage are:
- a protective (cotton) sleeve to protect the skin;
- cotton wool is used as an second layer and for padding (in MCB) or as padding alone (in MLB);
- multiple layers of short stretch bandages are applied on top of the cotton wool or cotton sleeve with padding.

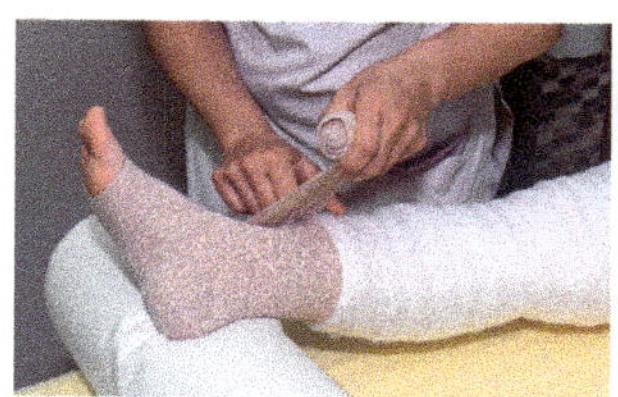
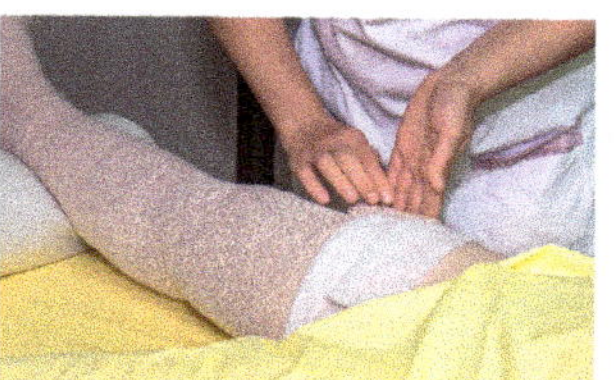
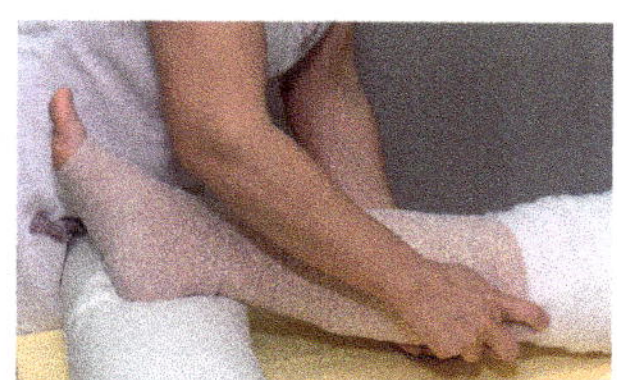

Figure 7.9 Multiple layers of short stretch bandages.

Alternative compression systems to short stretch are:

- 2-component self-adhesive compression systems;
- Velcro adjustable compression systems.

2-component compression systems

2-component compression systems have a self-adhesive component. The most common systems are Coban and Coflex. Coban has a self-adhesive comfort and compression layer, while Coflex only has a self-adhesive compression layer. These types of compression systems were primarily developed for the treatment of venous ulcers. Studies have demonstrated that these compression systems can also be incorporated in edema therapy, as well.[32-34] In comparison with short stretch bandaging, the 2-component systems are more expensive (and should therefore be discussed with the patient). 2-component systems stay in place for 3 to 4 days. The treatment effect of changing a 2-component system once every 3 days is equally effective as reapplying a short stretch bandage once daily. 2-component systems can help in decreasing the therapy time for the patients as well as the PT.

Figure 7.11 shows a comparison between the sub-bandage pressure of Coban and Coflex. A short stretch bandage was applied as well. Stiffness was also calculated.

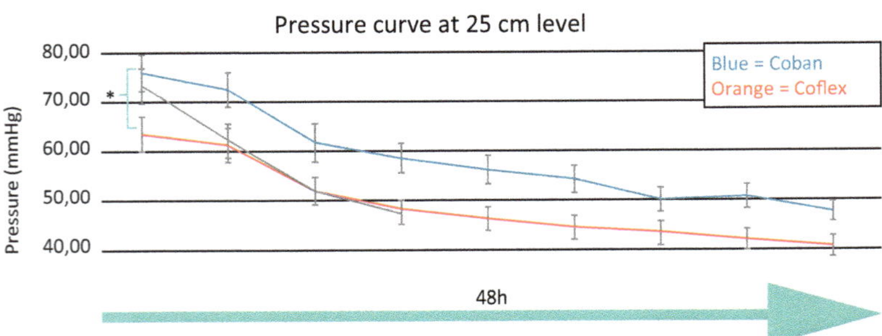

*Coban, Coflex, short stretch; * significant difference.*

Figure 7.10 Pressure curve of 2-component compression systems over 48h.

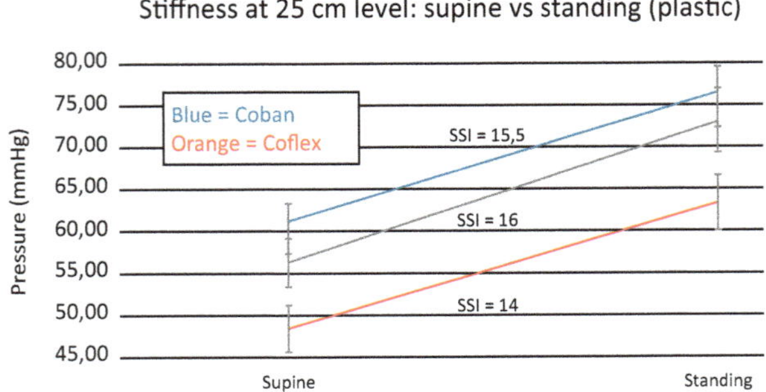

Figure 7.11 SSI from supine to standing position.

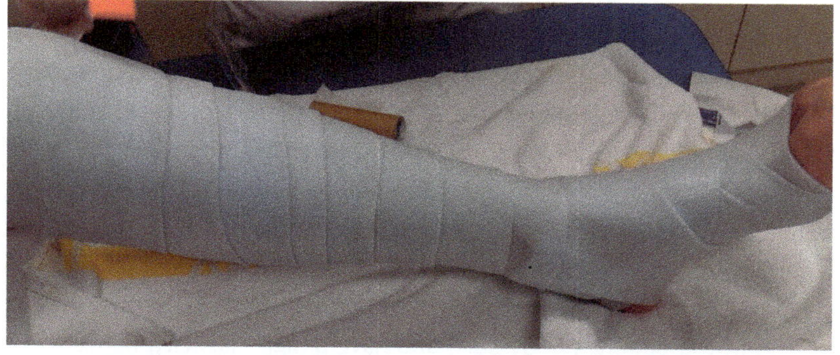

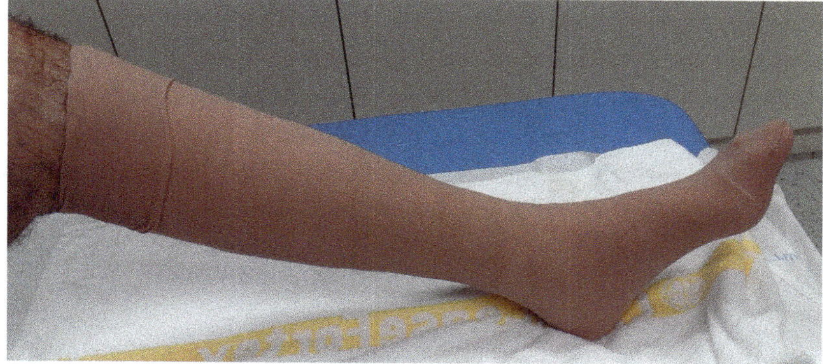

 Application of a 2-component compression system (CoFlex TLC). The first photo shows the comfort layer and the second photo shows the finished compression system, with the compression layer and nylon stocking in place. The nylon stocking is used to avoid creep of clothing and makes it easier to put on shoes.

Velcro adjustable compression systems

Velcro adjustable compression systems like the Circaid juxtafit can also be used. The Velcro system enables the continuous adjustment of the sub-bandage pressure, and this can easily be done by the patient him/herself. Circaid is often implemented as an adjuvant therapy in the maintenance phase if garments tend to be insufficient. Again, this is an expensive tool to be financed by the patient.

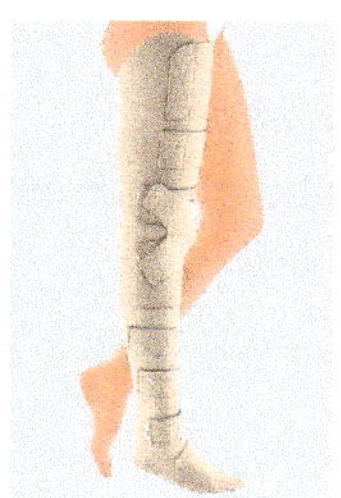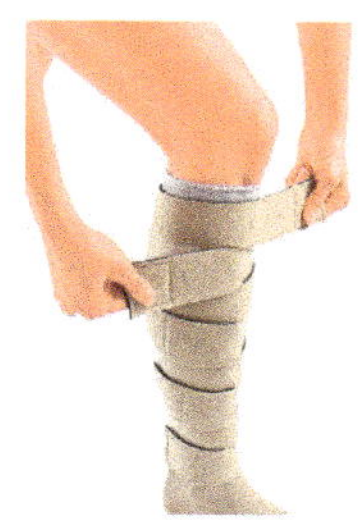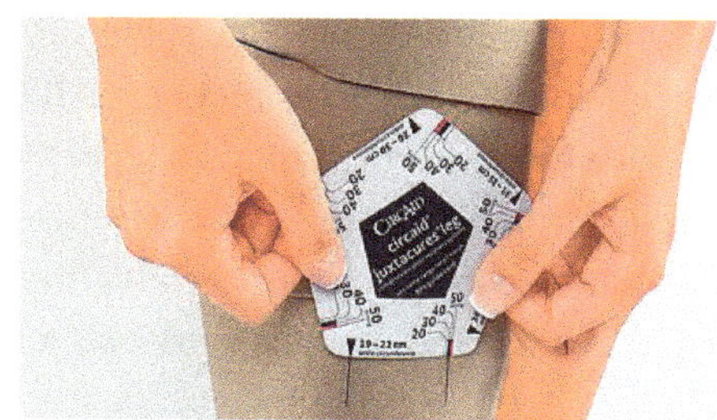

Source: Circaid® Juxtafit®; www.medi.nl

 Circaid® Juxtafit® Velcro compression system.

During the second phase of CDT (maintenance phase), bandages are most often replaced by compression garments. Compression garments provide a force against swelling and will not decrease the edema volume any further. In daily practice, compression garments are sometimes provided to patients with pitting edema in the belief that compression garments are able to decrease edema volume. This belief is false; physicians and patients should be informed properly about the correct application of compression therapy. Another common mistake is that round knit garments are a good compression modality for treating lymphedema. Round knit fabrics are off the shelf (they more or less fit the patient's body part) and have a high elasticity, hence a low stiffness and are therefore less suitable for edema therapy. Due to the high elasticity a round knit garment will still allow some additional swelling. Again, this is important information for health-care workers involved in the treatment of patients with chronic edema. It is also important that the patient is informed about the disadvantages of round knit garments. Many patients will have already worn round knit garments and will complain about how uncomfortable they are (which they are indeed).

Remark:
Imagine what happens when you put a rubber band around your fingers and you then try to open your fingers. Indeed, it will be possible to open your fingers despite the tight feeling of the elastic band. The same is possible when round knit stockings are worn by patients; they experience a tight feeling, yet the stocking will give way if swelling increases.

A different and more appropriate technology for producing garments is called flat knitting. Flat knit compression garments are less elastic in comparison to round knit garments. They are stiffer and will allow significantly less creep than round knit garments. This is because flat knit garments are most often custom made, based on a detailed measurement of the patient's body part. The working mechanism of a flat knit compression garment is two-fold:

- First, the garment will produce some sub-bandage pressure, increasing the tissue pressure and consequently limiting net filtration from the microcirculation.
- Second, when fluid starts to build up in the interstitial area, the sub-bandage pressure will further increase significantly (due to high stiffness and low creep).
- Next, the fluid is evacuated towards the proximal part of the garment (Pascal's Law), towards an area with a better working lymphatic system.

Round knit compression fabrics	Flat knit compression fabrics
Tubular knitting technology	Flat knitting starts from one piece of flat fabric → custom-made based on the measurements of the patient's body part → sewed into a tubular shape
High elasticity coefficient/Low to moderate stiffness	Low elasticity/high stiffness
No/ limited control of sub-bandage pressure	Controlled sub-bandage pressure (gradient)
Phlebological conditions	Lymphedema
No seam	A seam is often visible

Table 7.4   Main differences between round and flat knit fabrics.

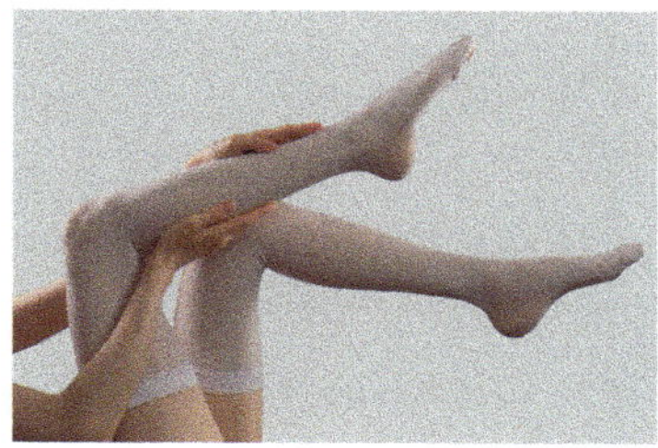
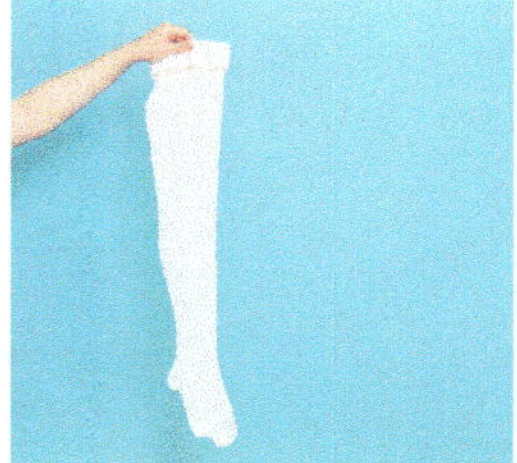

Figure 7.14   Compression stockings as an example of round knit compression fabrics.

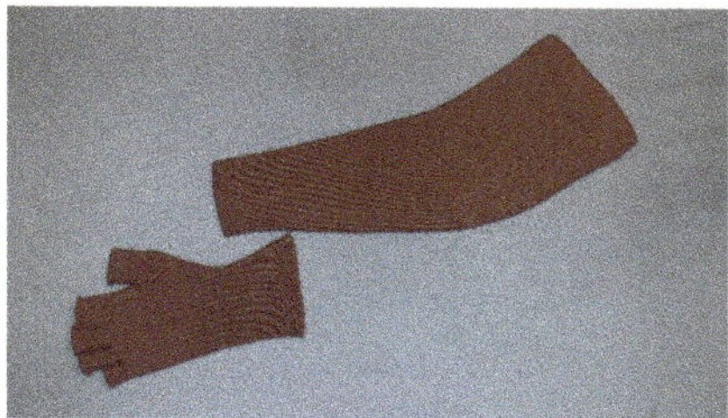

Figure 7.15   An example of flat knit compression fabrics.

To achieve the most effective treatment result, it is important that the garments are constructed when there is no longer any pitting present. It is preferable for the garments to be discussed in close collaboration between the patient, physical therapist and medical supplier. The medical supplier is responsible for the measurements and the custom-made fabrication of the garments. However, the feedback from the patient as well as the PT can be of great importance in deciding how the garment needs to be made. Since most patients achieve the leanest volume in the morning it would be best if the measurement is taken as early in the day as possible. Additionally, treatment needs to be continued until the garments have been produced and are available to the patient. The medical supplier trains the patient (and care providers) in the correct application of the garments. This is a very important part of the maintenance phase. If patients are unable to put on or take off the garments, they will not wear the garments.

Therefore, training them as well as caregivers is essential; if necessary the additional use of donning aids needs to be discussed (see the section on donning aid below).

Garments can be made for almost every part of the body. The most common garments are stockings (AD = knee height or AG = groin height), sleeves and gloves. The most common types of compression are displayed in table 7.5.

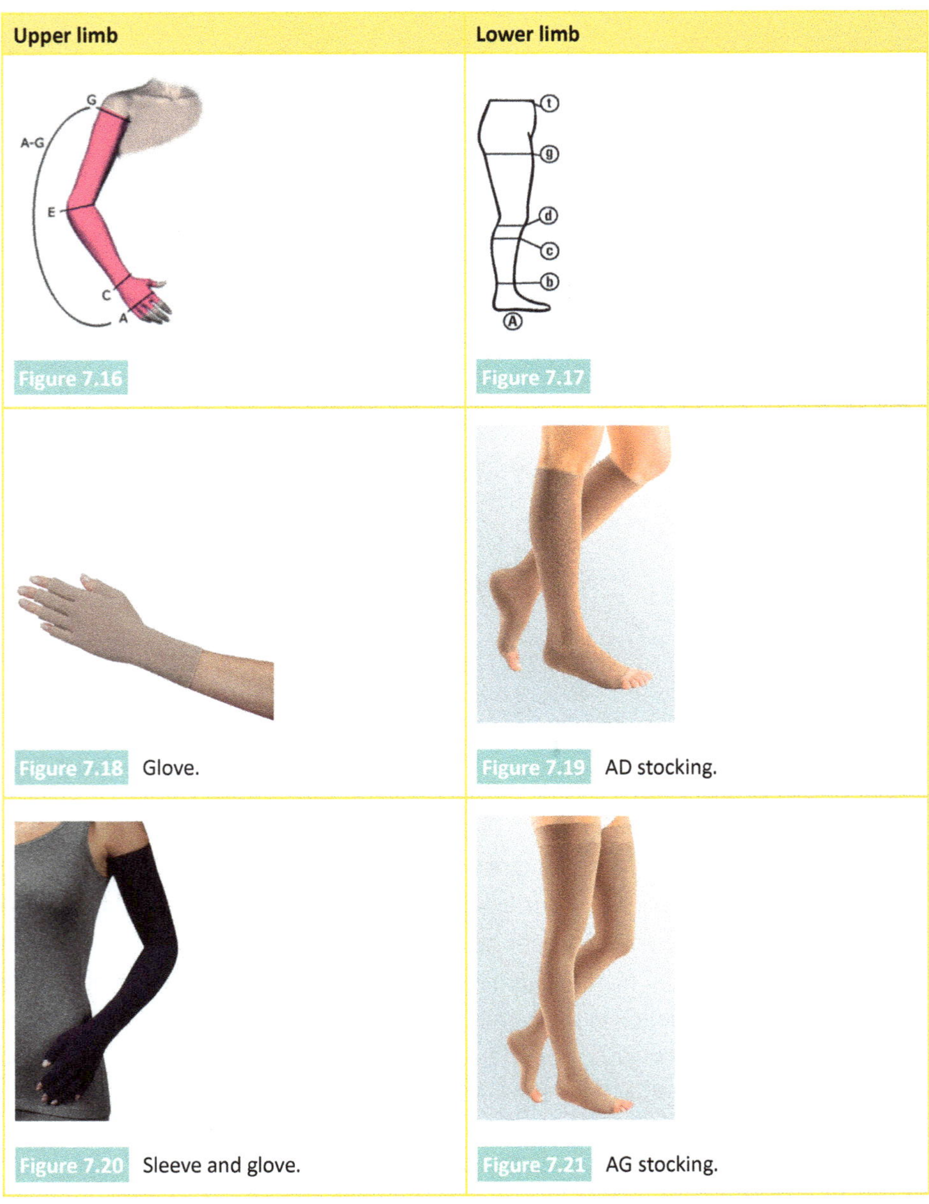

Upper limb	Lower limb
Figure 7.16	Figure 7.17
Figure 7.18 Glove.	Figure 7.19 AD stocking.
Figure 7.20 Sleeve and glove.	Figure 7.21 AG stocking.

Table 7.5 Overview of common compression garments for the upper and lower limb.

Compression garments are constructed based on compression classes. It is important to know that reimbursement can depend on the type of compression (round versus flat knit), compression class (I-IV) and the pathology. Accordingly, it is important to inform the patient about reimbursement policies. This is also the responsibility of the medical supplier and the referring physician who needs to provide the correct prescription. As both the physician and the medical supplier only see the patient occasionally, many patients will ask their physical therapist for information.

Another point of attention is the difference between countries (areas) with respect to the compression classes. The review of Palfreyman and Michaels provides a good overview of these differences (table 7.6).[35]

	Sub-bandage pressure range (mmHg)			
	Class 1	Class 2	Class 3	Class 4
British standard	14-17	18-24	25-35	N/A
German standard	18-21	23-32	34-46	> 49
French standard	10-15	15-20	20-36	> 36
Draft European standard	15-21	23-32	34-46	> 49
USA standard	15-20	20-30	30-40	N/A

Table 7.6 Differences between countries.[35]

Donning aid

Putting on compression garments can be difficult for patients, especially for patients with comorbidities on the musculoskeletal level, older patients and patients with movement restrictions. This difficulty can also increase along with the compression class. Several donning aids are available which can help to reduce the burden and increase compliance. Most frequently, a compression stocking comes with an easy slide fabric. This donning aid will reduce the resistance of the skin and help slip the compression stocking in place. Additionally, rubber gloves can be used by the patient to apply more force in donning the compression garment. Butler aids can be provided as well; these frames with handlebars allow the patient to drape the stocking or sleeve on the butler and use the handlebars to put on the stocking (figure 7.22). This type of donning aid is also available for sleeves.

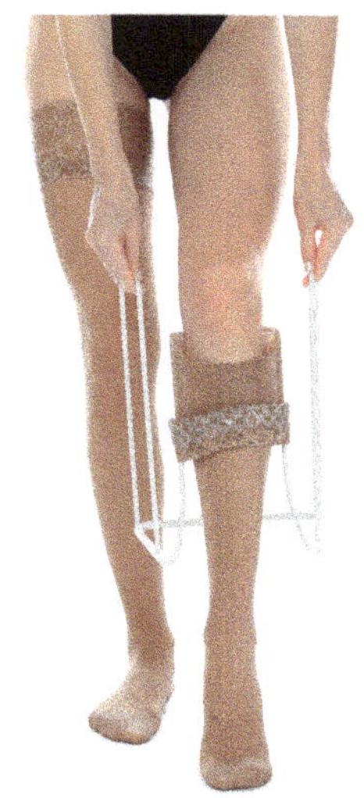

Figure 7.22 Example of a butler donning aid for lower limb compression stockings

7.2.4 Exercise therapy

Exercise is extremely important in edema therapy. The aim of exercising is to:
- stimulate and improve lymph flow (by increased muscle pumping and breathing frequency);
- stimulate lymphangiogenesis (new formation of lymphatics);
- awake 'sleeping' lymphatics (collateral vessels);
- promote/increase general health and limit the risk of edema exacerbations.

Exercising during edema therapy is again defined based on the two phases of Complex Decongestive Therapy (CDT).

During the **first phase** of CDT, breathing exercises can be implemented during the execution of the MLD maneuvers or during bandaging. Enhanced breathing will create much higher abdominal and thorax pressure changes, improving the lymph flow within the thoracic duct and other trunks as well.

Other exercises are provided after the compression bandages are in place. It is important to exercise with the compression system in place, since the muscle activities (contractions) will also create pressure changes underneath the bandage and stimulate the epifascial lymphatics. If possible, patients should do multiple short bouts of 10-15 minutes of exercise multiple times a day. This is important to discuss with the patient because they should exercise on their own and not only in the PT practice. Provide them with sufficiently detailed exercise schemes. Apart from the exercises that address the muscles of the edematous limb, it is also important to include general physical activities like walking, cycling and swimming (also with compression on). Try to find out which kind of activities are interesting to the patient. Patients will be more and longer motivated if they can perform activities that they like instead of dictated activities/exercises. It is important to start with a supervised protocol in order to guide, inform and correct the execution of exercises. Again, since exercising is the responsibility of the patients, progression should be made from supervised to a non-supervised protocol.

In **phase two** of CDT, the aim of exercise is to restore and improve physical endurance and to facilitate the participation in sports. An important message that needs to be discussed with the patients is the safety of sports and resistance training. As mentioned earlier, movement of the skin, muscle pumping and increased breathing are all stimuli that benefit increased lymph flow. However, for many years, patients with lymphedema or at risk of developing lymphedema were told to take more rest and to limit their amount of strenuous activities. The fact that these beliefs are still impacting the knowledge of patients about lymphedema was clearly demonstrated by a study conducted by Lee et al. in 2009 (13 years after the first results that demonstrated that exercise is beneficial and not harmful for patients with chronic edema). In a survey on 175 breast cancer patients, 70% replied that they avoided strenuous activity because they thought it would be increase the risk of or exacerbate lymphedema.[36]

Already in 1996, the first results from the dragon boat project (Harris, Canada) were published to tackle the myth about avoiding resistance training in lymphedema patients.[37] Since then, evidence has strengthened that exercising and sports are harmless and completely safe for patients with lymphedema. A systematic review published in 2011 concluded: "**Resistance training, taking into account a steady progression, is safe and does not increase edema burden; on the contrary, several beneficial effects are provoked**".[38] Physical therapists are ideally trained to instruct, guide and empower patients in exercise therapy and the resumption of sports.

What the physiotherapist needs to know:
- The conservative treatment of chronic edema is a combination therapy that includes at least the pillars of skin care, compression therapy and exercises.
- The conservative treatment can be broadened with additional pillars like MLD, diet and psychological support.
- The conservative treatment has two distinct phases with different aims. The intensive treatment phase is used to decrease the edema volume, while the maintenance phase is used to control the edema volume and increase physical endurance and functionality in daily life.
- Patients with chronic edema should be encouraged to move frequently; aerobic exercises are beneficial as are resistance trainings.
- Flat knit compression garments are most often provided to patients with chronic edema. A compression garment should not be the first type of therapy (unless provided as prevention in a non-swollen limb).

What other health-care professionals need to know:
- Although chronic edema is a symptom of an underlying aetiology, the edema can be treated. No patient should receive the news that they should learn to live with it.
- The earlier treatment is started, the higher the success rate; accordingly, if chronic edema is seen by other health-care professionals they should refer these patients to edema therapy specialists as soon as possible.
- Do not recommend compression garments as treatment for limbs that are actually swollen. Compression garments are not designed to reduce the edema volume, they are designed to maintain (control) the edema volume reduction.

- While compression garments work well in the maintenance phase, many patients are reluctant to wear them appropriately. It is therefore important that health-care professionals emphasize the importance of compression garments to patients with chronic edema.
- Motivate patients with chronic edema to be physically active, as muscle pumping facilitates lymphatic flow.

7.3 REFERENCES

1. The diagnosis and treatment of peripheral lymphedema: 2020 Consensus Document of the International Society of Lymphology. Lymphology. 2020;53(1):3-19.
2. Damstra RJ, Halk AB. The Dutch lymphedema guidelines based on the International Classification of Functioning, Disability, and Health and the chronic care model. J Vasc Surg Venous Lymphat Disord. 2017;5(5):756-765.
3. Halk AB, Damstra RJ. First Dutch guidelines on lipedema using the international classification of functioning, disability and health. Phlebology. 2017;32(3):152-159.
4. Gebruers N, Verbelen H, De Vrieze T, et al. Current and future perspectives on the evaluation, prevention and conservative management of breast cancer related lymphoedema: A best practice guideline. European journal of obstetrics, gynecology, and reproductive biology. 2017;216:245-253.
5. Gebruers N, Camberlin M, Theunissen F, et al. The effect of training interventions on physical performance, quality of life, and fatigue in patients receiving breast cancer treatment: a systematic review. Supportive care in cancer: official journal of the Multinational Association of Supportive Care in Cancer. 2019;27(1):109-122.
6. Asdourian MS, Skolny MN, Brunelle C, Seward CE, Salama L, Taghian AG. Precautions for breast cancer-related lymphoedema: risk from air travel, ipsilateral arm blood pressure measurements, skin puncture, extreme temperatures, and cellulitis. Lancet Oncol. 2016;17(9):e392-405.
7. Jones A, Woods M, Malhotra K. Critical examination of skin care self-management in lymphoedema. British journal of community nursing. 2019;24(Sup10):S6-s10.
8. Rich A. How to care for uncomplicated skin and keep it free of complications. British journal of community nursing. 2007;12(4):S6-9.
9. Woods M. Care of skin that is oedematous or at risk of oedema. Br J Nurs. 2019;28(11):674-676.
10. Fife CE, Farrow W, Hebert AA, et al. Skin and Wound Care in Lymphedema Patients: A Taxonomy, Primer, and Literature Review. Adv Skin Wound Care. 2017;30(7):305-318.
11. Bosompra K, Ashikaga T, O'Brien PJ, Nelson L, Skelly J, Beatty DJ. Knowledge about preventing and managing lymphedema: a survey of recently diagnosed and treated breast cancer patients. Patient education and counseling. 2002;47(2):155-163.
12. Tambour M, Holt M, Speyer A, Christensen R, Gram B. Manual lymphatic drainage adds no further volume reduction to Complete Decongestive Therapy on breast cancer-related lymphoedema: a multicentre, randomised, single-blind trial. Br J Cancer. 2018;119(10):1215-1222.
13. Gradalski T, Ochalek K, Kurpiewska J. Complex Decongestive Lymphatic Therapy With or Without Vodder II Manual Lymph Drainage in More Severe Chronic Postmastectomy Upper Limb Lymphedema: A Randomized Noninferiority Prospective Study. J Pain Symptom Manage. 2015;50(6):750-757.
14. Bergmann A, da Costa Leite Ferreira MG, de Aguiar SS, et al. Physiotherapy in upper limb lymphedema after breast cancer treatment: a randomized study. Lymphology. 2014;47(2):82-91.
15. Ezzo J, Manheimer E, McNeely ML, et al. Manual lymphatic drainage for lymphedema following breast cancer treatment. The Cochrane database of systematic reviews. 2015(5):Cd003475.
16. Liang M, Chen Q, Peng K, et al. Manual lymphatic drainage for lymphedema in patients after breast cancer surgery: A systematic review and meta-analysis of randomized controlled trials. Medicine (Baltimore). 2020;99(49):e23192.

17.   Huang TW, Tseng SH, Lin CC, et al. Effects of manual lymphatic drainage on breast cancer-related lymphedema: a systematic review and meta-analysis of randomized controlled trials. World journal of surgical oncology. 2013;11:15.

18.   Devoogdt N, Geraerts I, Van Kampen M, et al. Manual lymph drainage may not have a preventive effect on the development of breast cancer-related lymphoedema in the long term: a randomised trial. Journal of physiotherapy. 2018;64(4):245-254.

19.   Torres Lacomba M, Yuste Sanchez MJ, Zapico Goni A, et al. Effectiveness of early physiotherapy to prevent lymphoedema after surgery for breast cancer: randomised, single blinded, clinical trial. BMJ (Clinical research ed). 2010;340:b5396.

20.   Baumann FT, Bloch W, Weissen A, et al. Physical Activity in Breast Cancer Patients during Medical Treatment and in the Aftercare – a Review. Breast Care. 2013;8(5):330-334.

21.   De Vrieze T, Vos L, Gebruers N, et al. Protocol of a randomised controlled trial regarding the effectiveness of fluoroscopy-guided manual lymph drainage for the treatment of breast cancer-related lymphoedema (EFforT-BCRL trial). European journal of obstetrics, gynecology, and reproductive biology. 2018;221:177-188.

22.   Belgrado JP, Vandermeeren L, Vankerckhove S, et al. Near-Infrared Fluorescence Lymphatic Imaging to Reconsider Occlusion Pressure of Superficial Lymphatic Collectors in Upper Extremities of Healthy Volunteers. Lymphat Res Biol. 2016.

23.   Vignes S, Porcher R, Arrault M, Dupuy A. Long-term management of breast cancer-related lymphedema after intensive decongestive physiotherapy. Breast cancer research and treatment. 2007;101(3):285-290.

24.   Vignes S, Porcher R, Arrault M, Dupuy A. Factors influencing breast cancer-related lymphedema volume after intensive decongestive physiotherapy. Supportive care in cancer: official journal of the Multinational Association of Supportive Care in Cancer. 2011;19(7):935-940.

25.   Hettrick. The Science of Compression Therapy for Chronic Venous Insufficiency Edema. Journal of the American College of Certified Wound Specialists. 2009;1:20-24.

26.   Partsch H. The static stiffness index: a simple method to assess the elastic property of compression material in vivo. Dermatol Surg. 2005;31(6):625-630.

27.   Partsch H. Compression therapy: clinical and experimental evidence. Ann Vasc Dis. 2012;5(4):416-422.

28.   Partsch H, Schuren J, Mosti G, Benigni JP. The Static Stiffness Index: an important parameter to characterise compression therapy in vivo. J Wound Care. 2016;25 Suppl 9:S4-s10.

29.   Hirai M, Niimi K, Iwata H, et al. Comparison of stiffness and interface pressure during rest and exercise among various arm sleeves. Phlebology. 2010;25(4):196-200.

30.   Damstra RJ, Brouwer ER, Partsch H. Controlled, comparative study of relation between volume changes and interface pressure under short-stretch bandages in leg lymphedema patients. Dermatol Surg. 2008;34(6):773-778; discussion 778-779.

31.   Partsch H, Damstra RJ, Mosti G. Dose finding for an optimal compression pressure to reduce chronic edema of the extremities. International angiology: a journal of the International Union of Angiology. 2011;30(6):527-533.

32.   Franks PJ, Moffatt CJ, Murray S, Reddick M, Tilley A, Schreiber A. Evaluation of the performance of a new compression system in patients with lymphoedema. Int Wound J. 2013;10(2):203-209.

33.   Moffatt CJ, Franks PJ, Hardy D, Lewis M, Parker V, Feldman JL. A preliminary randomized controlled study to determine the application frequency of a new lymphoedema bandaging system. Br J Dermatol. 2012;166(3):624-632.

34.   Torres-Lacomba M, Navarro-Brazález B, Prieto-Gómez V, Ferrandez JC, Bouchet JY, Romay-Barrero H. Effectiveness of four types of bandages and kinesio-tape for treating breast-cancer-related lymphoedema: a randomized, single-blind, clinical trial. Clinical rehabilitation. 2020;34(9):1230-1241.

35.   Palfreyman SJ, Michaels JA. A systematic review of compression hosiery for uncomplicated varicose veins. Phlebology. 2009;24 Suppl 1:13-33.

36.   Lee TS, Kilbreath SL, Sullivan G, Refshauge KM, Beith JM. Patient perceptions of arm care and exercise advice after breast cancer surgery. Oncol Nurs Forum. 2010;37(1):85-91.

37.   Harris SR. "We're All in the Same Boat": A Review of the Benefits of Dragon Boat Racing for Women Living with Breast Cancer. Evid Based Complement Alternat Med. 2012;2012:167651.

38.   Kwan ML, Cohn JC, Armer JM, Stewart BR, Cormier JN. Exercise in patients with lymphedema: a systematic review of the contemporary literature. J Cancer Surviv. 2011;5(4):320-336.

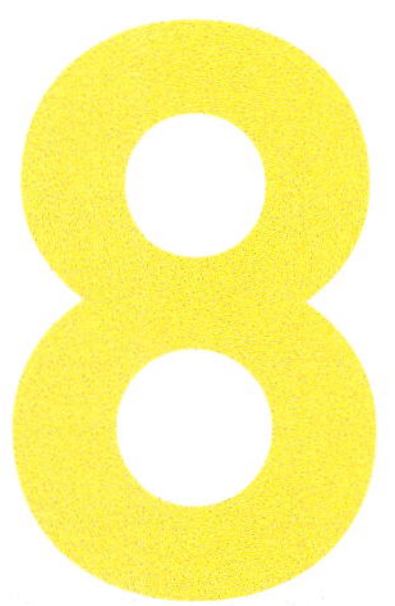

8 MANAGEMENT OF BREAST EDEMA

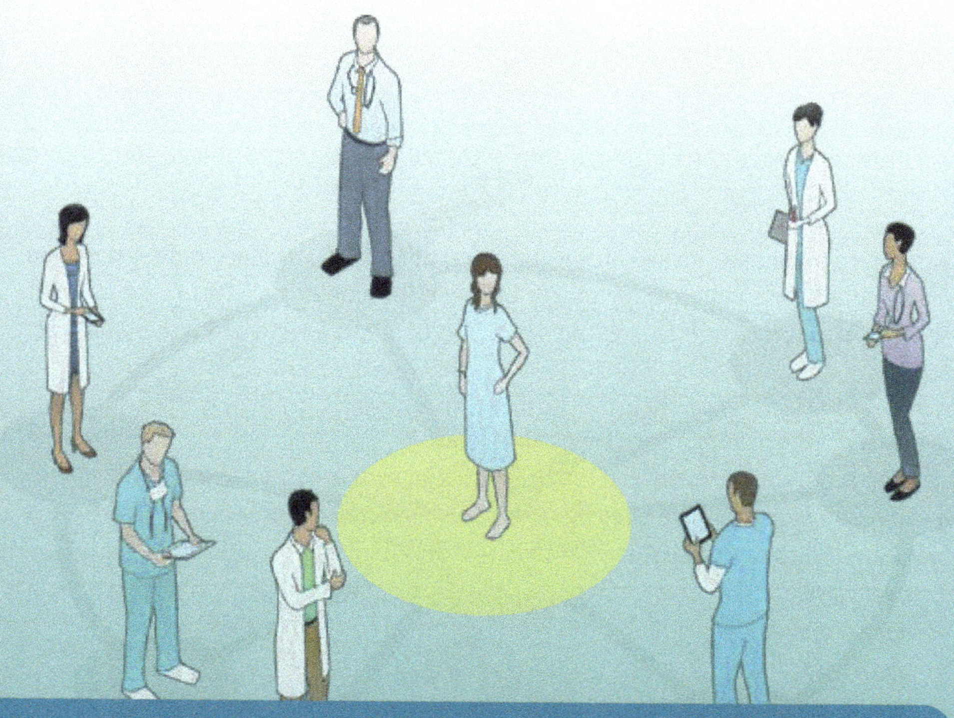

The learning objectives for this chapter are:
- Providing insight into the aetiology of breast edema
- Identifying the assessment methods of breast edema
- Describing the longitudinal course of breast edema
- Obtaining an approach to treating breast edema

8.1   INTRODUCTION

Breast conserving surgery (BCS) followed by radiotherapy is a safe and effective procedure for treating patients with early stage breast cancer. However, some patients will
be troubled by breast edema in the operated and irradiated breast. Breast edema is far
less explored in literature compared to lymphedema of the arm, but it is gaining rele-
vance due to the increase in patients receiving BCS together with adjuvant radiotherapy. Both aspects of this treatment can cause breast edema. The surgery itself can cause
damage to the lymphatic system, which can lead to a compromised transport capacity
not only in the arm, but also in the breast. However, the main contributing factor is
radiotherapy, which causes various tissue reactions, including edema.[1]

8.2   WHAT IS BREAST EDEMA?

8.2.1   Definition

Based on a systematic review of the literature, the overall incidence of breast edema
following BCS and radiotherapy ranges between 0% and 90.4%.[2] This range includes
all kinds of assessment methods and definitions of breast edema and is therefore very
broad.

In breast edema patients, breast size can increase by more than one cup size. However,
swelling is not the only criterion that is associated with breast edema and sometimes
it can occur without visible swelling. The following diagnostic criteria are found in the
literature, which can present in many different ways:
- swelling;
- peau d'orange;
- hardness;
- heaviness;
- redness;
- pain;
- tensed skin;
- pitting.

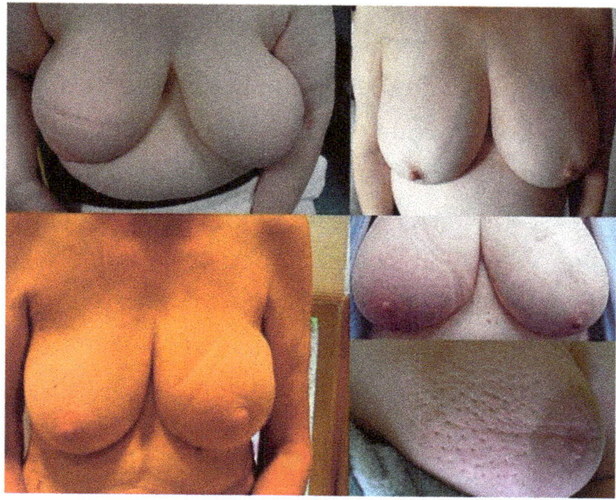

Figure 8.1   Visible signs of breast edema: pitting, swelling, peau d'orange.

8.2.2   Stages of breast edema

Breast edema can be divided into different stages.
- Stage 1 is characterized by a thickening of the skin, while the breast volume remains unchanged.
- In stage 2, breast edema presents as a visible edema which can lead to asymmetry between both breasts. In patients with severe breast edema, the volume of the operated and irradiated breast can sometimes increase up to 300 ml. Stage 2 is further characterized by dilated skin pores (referred to as peau d'orange), heaviness, pain and pitting edema on the affected breast.
- Stage 3 of breast edema is similar to stage 2, but in this stage the pain is more extensive.[3]

8.2.3   Components of breast edema

Wratten et al. describe two components of breast edema:
- Firstly, generalized enlargement or swelling of the breast tissue itself may occur, which is referred to as parenchymal breast edema.
- Secondly, there may be evidence of edematous changes in the epidermis and dermis, which is referred to as cutaneous breast edema. Although cutaneous breast edema may occur by itself, in many instances there will be a combination of both components.[4]

8.3 ASSESSMENT OF BREAST EDEMA

A rigorous systematic review was published in 2014 on the topic of breast edema found that a standardized protocol for assessing breast edema as well as a clear definition for diagnosis was lacking.[2] A physical examination is the most commonly used method found in the literature for assessing breast edema, with symptoms of breast edema being evaluated by means of inspection, palpation and anamnesis.[5-16] Additionally, clinical pictures of the breasts can be taken in order to assess the evolution more accurately.[17-19] Furthermore, several imaging techniques are described in the literature, including high-frequency ultrasound (HFUS). Clinical signs of breast edema on HFUS are a thickening of the skin greater than 2 mm with increased echogenicity, disturbance or poor visibility of the deeper echogenic line and interstitial fluid accumulation.[6,20,21] An MRI makes it possible to detect fluid-containing formations such as parenchymal and cutaneous breast edema, which are visible as white areas.[22] Using mammography, parenchymal breast edema is seen as trabecular thickening and cutaneous breast edema as skin thickening.[23] Another technique that can provide information on breast edema is tissue dielectric current (TDC), which is measured using the MoistureMeterD. This device can measure local tissue water to the depth of 2.5mm or 5mm. A TDC ratio between the affected and healthy breast that is equal to or greater than 1.40 is considered to be breast edema.[24]

As a result of the different definitions and assessment methods used, breast edema incidence range is very broad.[2] With this conclusion in mind, the Breast Edema Questionnaire (BrEQ) was developed.[25] This Dutch questionnaire is the first such questionnaire for assessing breast edema in breast cancer patients with evidence of validity and reliability. Furthermore, the synthesis of symptoms listed in the BrEQ can serve as a catalyst for developing a standard definition for breast edema. In the first part of the questionnaire, symptoms of breast edema are scored on a scale from 0 to 10: pain, heaviness, swelling, tensed skin, redness, pitting sign, enlarged skin pores and hardness. Taking into account the International Classification of Functioning, Disability and Health (ICF), several activity limitations and participation restrictions are scored from 0 to 10 in part 2. Clinimetric properties of the BrEQ were tested in a group of breast cancer patients who underwent BCS and radiotherapy. This test found that the BrEQ is a reliable and valid Dutch questionnaire for assessing breast edema and its impact on daily functioning. Moreover, for part 1 of the BrEQ, a score cut-off point of 8.5 is determined. A BrEQ score of 9 or higher discriminates between patients who have breast edema and those who have not.[25] In conclusion, the BrEQ is a useful tool for assessing and diagnosing breast edema in clinical practice and gaining insight into its impact on daily functioning.

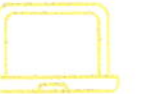

The BrEQ-questionnaire can be found on the online learning platform Sofia.

8.4 LONGITUDINAL COURSE

Several studies investigated the natural course of breast edema over time and demonstrated similar findings.[8,11,15,24,26,27] Table 8.1 provides an overview of the available literature in which all assessment methods and all definitions of breast edema are included. In female breast cancer patients who underwent BCS in combination with radiotherapy, a peak in prevalence was observed after termination of radiotherapy. Afterwards, a gradual spontaneous decline can be expected in the following months.[28]

Reference	Follow-up	Breast edema prevalence
Verbelen (own data, not published)	Prior to RT After termination of RT 3 months after RT 6 months after RT 12 months after RT	52.5% 63.8% 55.3% 57.1% 47.5%
Adriaenssens 2012[26]	0-3 months postoperative 3-6 months postoperative 6-12 months postoperative 12-24 months postoperative 24-60 months postoperative	93.3% 73.3% 82.4% 80.6% 65.4%
Berrang 2011[11]	Prior to RT 1 year after RT 3 years after RT	32% 16% 6%
Vicini 2007[8]	> 6 months after RT > 24 months after RT > 36 months after RT	32% 22% 0%
Young-Afat 2019[27]	Baseline: prior to RT 3 months after baseline 6 months after baseline 12 months after baseline 18 months after baseline	12.0% 7.1% 12.4% 8.2% 5.5%
Olivotto 1996[15]	Prior to RT 3 year after RT 5 years after RT	26.6% 4.3% 2.6%
Johansson 2015[24]	Prior to RT 2 weeks after RT 3 months after RT 6 months after RT 12 months after RT 24 months after RT	29% 39% 63% 63% 39% 28%
Lam 2020[29] (meta-analysis)	0-4 weeks after RT 6 months-10 years after RT	26.2%-47.1% 7.2%-9.9%

Abbreviations: RT: radiation therapy.
Most studies, apart from Adriaenssens et al., are based on the timing of RT to describe the time course of breast edema. Data concerning the amount of time postoperatively is not available.
Source: Based on the findings of Lam 2020 (a meta-analysis), about 7-10% of the patients will need treatment for breast edema provoked by BCS and radiotherapy.

Table 8.1   Time course of breast edema in the scientific literature.

The degree of breast edema has about the same timeline as its prevalence. Few studies have investigated its degree longitudinally. Wratten et al. described the time course of cutaneous breast edema based on the increase in epidermal thickness, measured with US. In most breast cancer patients who underwent BCS and radiotherapy, epidermal thickness usually peaks at 4 to 6 months post-treatment and in most instances show signs of returning to baseline 12 months post-treatment. The course of parenchymal breast edema has about the same timeline.[20]

In many patients, breast edema is already present prior to radiotherapy. This can be explained by several factors:

- First, the fact that BCS itself causes breast edema, due to damage to the lymphatic system. This compromises lymphatic transport and could therefore cause breast edema.[2]
- Second, after BCS, breast edema could be mistaken for typical postoperative complaints, such as pain, swelling and tensed skin, which are not in fact directly associated with breast edema.

A spontaneous decline in breast edema symptoms within 6 months after termination of radiotherapy is referred to as transient breast edema. In if the breast symptoms show no signs of returning to normal more than 6 months post-radiation, it is referred to as persistent breast edema. We strongly advise patients and health-care workers involved in the treatment and after-treatment of breast cancer patients to closely monitor breast complaints after radiotherapy. In cases of mild breast symptoms and/or transient breast edema, no treatment is necessary. Patients with persistent breast edema and/or patients in whom the breast complaints are very pronounced and bothersome are recommended to pursue appropriate treatment.

8.5 CONSERVATIVE TREATMENT OF BREAST EDEMA

The current evidence-based treatment for lymphedema of all sorts is complex decongestive therapy (CDT), which is generally accepted as the consensus treatment.[30,31] However, some aspects of CDT, namely the manual lymphatic drainage (MLD), are up for debate.[32-38] Although the literature on the treatment of breast edema in specific is scarce, we recommend extrapolating CDT – which is thoroughly described for the extremities (see Chapter 7) – to breast edema as well, to the utmost extent. The following is a synopsis of the four pillars of CDT and, where applicable, its evidence for breast edema.

8.5.1 Skin care

The purpose of skin care is to maintain a healthy skin barrier. Damaged and dry skin can become an entry point for infection. Therefore, good skin hygiene, precautionary measures and wound prevention can reduce the risk of infection and possible worsening of the breast edema. Patients are instructed to wash their skin daily with neutral soaps, dry their skin thoroughly with attention for the inframammary fold and use low pH lotions and emollients. In addition, patients are recommended to take precautionary measures. Besides skin hygiene, recommendations supported by scientific evidence for lymphedema in general are as follows: avoid trauma, disinfect and treat wounds immediately, avoid sauna visits and seek medical help in case of skin changes.[31] Additional information given to the patients can be relevant as well, as certain risk factors have been shown to aggravate lymphedema. The recommendations for avoiding these risk factors rely on common sense: maintain or achieve a healthy/normal BMI, protect the skin from sunburn and wear appropriate clothing and bra.[31] For breast edema in particular, risk factors are investigated in a systematic review of the literature.[2] Table 8.2 provides an overview of the risk factors found in literature, though consensus among studies is lacking. Also, those risk factors are not likely to be reversible by actions of the patients.

Related to radiotherapy	• Increase in irradiated breast volume • Increase in boost volume • Photon boost • Increasing breast separation • External beam radiation (vs. intra-operative radiotherapy) • Conventional radiotherapy (vs. intensity-modulated radiotherapy)
Related to surgery	Postoperative infection
Related to tumour characteristics	Larger tumour
Related to personal factors	• Larger breast volume • Increasing breast density • Diabetes mellitus

Table 8.2 Risk factors for breast edema.

8.5.2 MLD

MLD is another pillar of CDT that can be performed during both the intensive phase and the maintenance phase. MLD is a massage technique that aims to promote the movement of lymphatic fluid out of the swollen area as well as the uptake of interstitial fluid by the lymphatic system.[39] Although MLD is a well-established treatment modality for lymphedema of the extremities in clinical practice, its effectiveness is still questioned among researchers.[32-38] For breast edema, scientific evidence concerning MLD is lacking, although it is often administered in clinical practice. Lymph fluid from the breast is drained proximally towards the axillary and supraclavicular lymph nodes and/or towards the lymph nodes of the contralateral side. Evidence needs to be established in order to determine whether or not MLD should be omitted definitively from CDT for breast edema. Nevertheless, pending evidence concerning the role of MLD, it is our current recommendation to exclude MLD from the breast edema treatment, as it is time consuming and costly.

8.5.3 Compression

During the intensive phase of CDT, compression (figure 8.2) is used in order to decrease the lymphedema volume, with short-stretch multilayer bandages most commonly used to provide this compression.[39] For breast edema, however, it is difficult to apply these bandages correctly and with the appropriate pressure and many women find them uncomfortable to wear. Therefore, a compression bra or sports bra of compression type can be provided instead. During the maintenance phase, the use of this type of bra can be continued. It is important to note that scientific evidence concerning compression therapy for women with breast edema is scarce. A study by Johansson et al. investigated the treatment of breast edema using a sports bra of compression type with firm pressure flattening the breasts and compared it with ordinary bras.[40] This type of compression needed to be worn during the daytime for 9 months. Results showed that this breast compression treatment had no effect on the symptoms of breast edema or on the amount of local tissue water measured by the TDC. Therefore, the recommendation is to wear a sports bra of compression type, only if it doesn't cause a negative impact on comfort. Additionally, closely monitor the symptoms of breast edema in order to intervene if necessary. Needless to say, more research on this topic is of great importance.

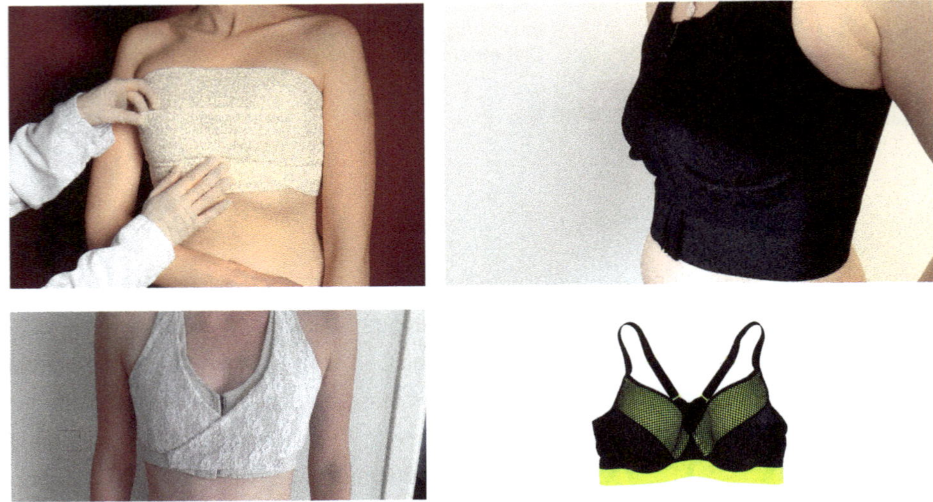

Figure 8.2   Compression of the breast by means of bandages, compression garment and sports bra.

8.5.4   Exercise

It has consistently been demonstrated that exercise is beneficial for managing lymph-edema, as well as aerobic exercise and resistance training. However, only one study has investigated whether women with breast edema would respond similarly to exercise than to those with arm edema.[41] This study investigated a supervised 12-week combined aerobic and resistance training programme. The exercise group reported a greater reduction in breast-related symptoms than the control group, assessed by the EORTC-BR23 breast symptom questions. Measures of extracellular fluid, assessed by means of bioimpedance spectroscopy ratio, decreased in the exercise group compared to the control group. No significant difference was detected in dermal thickness in the breast, assessed by ultrasound.[41] Improving the use of a muscle pump will stimulate the lymphatic transport, and improving the overall physical endurance and strength will lead to a better physical condition and coping.[31] Importantly, strenuous exercise will not aggravate the lymphedema, something which is often falsely assumed.[41,42] As such, exercise should not be avoided unless it provokes pain or articular problems.

What the physiotherapist needs to know:
- Patients treated with BCS and radiotherapy should be monitored until 12 months after the end of radiotherapy
- To aid in the detection and monitoring of breast edema, the use of the BrEQ in combination with a physical examination is a suitable approach.
- If no spontaneous decline of breast edema after 6 months is seen and no other treatable cause is found; start treating the edema.
- Currently, CDT, with the exception of MLD, is the recommended treatment, which involves skin care, compression and exercise therapy. However, strong scientific evidence for CDT still needs to be established.

What other health-care workers need to know:
- Patients should be informed about breast edema and its natural course.
- Patients should be monitored closely. If symptoms of breast edema occur, refer the patient to a specialized physiotherapist for appropriate treatment.

8.6 REFERENCES

1.   Kwak JY, Kim EK, Chung SY, You JK, Oh KK, Lee YH, et al. Unilateral breast edema: Spectrum of etiologies and imaging appearances. *Yonsei Med J.* 2005;46(1):1-7.

2.   Verbelen H, Gebruers N, Beyers T, De Monie A-C, Tjalma W. Breast edema in breast cancer patients following breast-conserving surgery and radiotherapy: a systematic review. *Breast Cancer Res Treat.* 2014;147(3).

3.   Delay E, Gosset J, Toussoun G, Delaporte T, Delbaere M. [Post-treatment sequelae after breast cancer conservative surgery]. *Ann Chir Plast esthétique.* 2008 Apr;53(2):135-52.

4.   Wratten CR, O'brien PC, Hamilton CS, Bill D, Kilmurray J, Denham JW. Breast edema in patients undergoing breast-conserving treatment for breast cancer: assessment via high frequency ultrasound. *Breast J.* 2007;13(3):266-73.

5.   Harsolia A, Kestin L, Grills I, Wallace M, Jolly S, Jones C, et al. Intensity-modulated radiotherapy results in significant decrease in clinical toxicities compared with conventional wedge-based breast radiotherapy. *Int J Radiat Oncol Biol Phys.* 2007 Aug;68(5):1375-80.

6.   Adriaenssens N, Belsack D, Buyl R, Ruggiero L, Breucq C, Mey J De, et al. Ultrasound elastography as an objective diagnostic measurement tool for lymphoedema of the treated breast in breast cancer patients following breast conserving surgery and radiotherapy. *Radiol. Oncol.* 2012;46(4):284-95.

7.   Goyal S, Daroui P, Khan AJ, Kearney T, Kirstein L, Haffty BG. Three-year outcomes of a once daily fractionation scheme for accelerated partial breast irradiation (APBI) using 3-D conformal radiotherapy (3D-CRT). *Cancer Med.* 2013;2(6):964-71.

8.   Vicini FA, Chen P, Wallace M, Mitchell C, Hasan Y, Grills I, Kestin L, Schell S, Goldstein NS, Kunzman J, Gilbert S, Martinez A. Interim cosmetic results and toxicity using 3D conformal external beam radiotherapy to deliver accelerated partial breast irradiation in patients with early-stage breast cancer treated with breast-conserving therapy. *Int J Radiat Oncol Biol Phys.* 2007 Nov 15;69(4):1124-30. doi: 10.1016/j.ijrobp.2007.04.033. PMID: 17967306.

9.   Chadha M, Vongtama D, Friedmann P, Parris C, Boolbol SK, Woode R, et al. Comparative Acute Toxicity from Whole Breast Irradiation Using 3-Week Accelerated Schedule With Concomitant Boost and the 6.5-Week Conventional Schedule With Sequential Boost for Early-Stage Breast Cancer. *Clin Breast Cancer.* 2012;12(1):57-62.

10.   Kelemen G, Varga Z, Lázár G, Thurzó L, Kahán Z. Cosmetic outcome 1-5 years after breast conservative surgery, irradiation and systemic therapy. *Pathol Oncol Res.* 2012;18(2):421-7.

11.   Berrang TS, Olivotto I, Kim D-H, Nichol A, Cho BCJ, Mohamed IG, et al. Three-year outcomes of a Canadian multicenter study of accelerated partial breast irradiation using conformal radiation therapy. *Int J Radiat Oncol Biol Phys.* 2011;81(5):1220-7.

12.   Mussari S, Sabino Della Sala W, Busana L, Vanoni V, Eccher C, Zani B, et al. Full-dose intraoperative radiotherapy with electrons in breast cancer. First report on late toxicity and cosmetic results from a single-institution experience. *Strahlenther Onkol.* 2006 Oct;182(10):589-95.

13.   Hoeller U, Tribius S, Kuhlmey A, Grader K, Fehlauer F, Alberti W. Increasing the rate of late toxicity by changing the score? A comparison of RTOG/EORTC and LENT/SOMA scores. *Int J Radiat Oncol Biol Phys.* 2003;55(4):1013-8.

14.   Grann A, McCormick B, Chabner ES, Gollamudi S V, Schupak KD, Mychalczak BR, et al. Prone breast radiotherapy in early-stage breast cancer: a preliminary analysis. *Int J Radiat Oncol.* 2000;47(2):319-25.

15.   Olivotto IA, Weir LM, Kim-Sing C, Bajdik CD, Trevisan CH, Doll CM, et al. Late cosmetic results of short fractionation for breast conservation. *Radiother Oncol.* 1996 Oct;41(1):7-13.

16.   Kuptsova N, Chang-Claude J, Kropp S, Helmbold I, Schmezer P, von Fournier D, et al. Genetic predictors of long-term toxicities after radiation therapy for breast cancer. *Int J Cancer.* 2008 Mar;122(6):1333-9.

17.   Toledano A, Garaud P, Serin D, Fourquet A, Bosset J-F, Breteau N, et al. Concurrent administration of adjuvant chemotherapy and radiotherapy after breast-conserving surgery enhances late toxicities: long-term results of the ARCOSEIN multicenter randomized study. *Int J Radiat Oncol Biol Phys.* 2006 Jun;65(2):324-32.

18. Barnett GC, Wilkinson JS, Moody AM, Wilson CB, Twyman N, Wishart GC, et al. The Cambridge Breast Intensity-modulated Radiotherapy Trial: Patient- and Treatment-related Factors that Influence Late Toxicity. *Clin Oncol.* 2011;23(10):662-73.

19. Marcenaro M, Sacco S, Pentimalli S, Berretta L, Andretta V, Grasso R, et al. Measures of late effects in conservative treatment of breast cancer with standard or hypofractionated radiotherapy. *Tumouri.* 2004;90(6):586-91.

20. Wratten CR, O'brien PC, Hamilton CS, Bill D, Kilmurray J, Denham JW. Breast edema in patients undergoing breast-conserving treatment for breast cancer: assessment via high frequency ultrasound. *Breast J.* 2007 May-Jun;13(3):266-73. doi: 10.1111/j.1524-4741.2007.00420.x. PMID: 17461901.

21. Wratten C, Kilmurray J, Wright S, O'Brien PC, Back M, Hamilton CS, Denham JW. Pilot study of high-frequency ultrasound to assess cutaneous oedema in the conservatively managed breast. *Int J Cancer.* 2000 Oct 20;90(5):295-301.

22. Forrai G, Polgar C, Zana K, Riedl E, Fodor J, Nemeth G, et al. The role of STIR MRI sequence in the evaluation of the breast following conservative surgery and radiotherapy. *Neoplasma.* 2001;48(1):7-11.

23. Kuzmiak CM, Zeng D, Cole E, Pisano ED. Mammographic Findings of Partial Breast Irradiation. *Acad Radiol.* 2009;16(7):819.

24. Johansson K, Darkeh MH, Lahtinen T, Björk-Eriksson T, Alexsson R. Two-year follow-up of temporal changes of breast edema after breast cancer treatment with surgery and radiation evaluated by tissue dielectric constant (TDC). *Eur J of Lymphol.* 2015;27(73):15-21.

25. Verbelen H, De Vrieze T, Van Soom T, Meirte J, Van Goethem M, Hufkens G, Tjalma W, Gebruers N. Development and clinimetric properties of the Dutch Breast Edema Questionnaire (BrEQ-Dutch version) to diagnose the presence of breast edema in breast cancer patients. *Qual Life Res.* 2020;29(2):569-578. doi: 10.1007/s11136-019-02337-z.

26. Adriaenssens N, Verbelen H, Lievens P, Lamote J. Lymphedema of the operated and irradiated breast in breast cancer patients following breast conserving surgery and radiotherapy. *Lymphology.* 2012 Dec;45(4):154-64.

27. Young-Afat DA, Gregorowitsch ML, van den Bongard DH, Burgmans I, van der Pol CC, Witkamp AJ, et al. Breast Edema Following Breast-Conserving Surgery and Radiotherapy: Patient-Reported Prevalence, Determinants, and Effect on Health-Related Quality of Life. *JNCI Cancer Spectr.* 2019;3(2):4-11.

28. Verbelen H. Arm, shoulder and breast morbidity after breast cancer treatment, PhD dissertation, University of Antwerp. 2020.

29. Lam E, Yee C, Wong G, Popovic M, Drost L, Pon K, et al. A systematic review and meta-analysis of clinician-reported versus patient-reported outcomes of radiation dermatitis. *Breast.* 2020; 50:125-34.

30. Executive Committee. The Diagnosis and Treatment of Peripheral Lymphedema: 2016 Consensus Document of the International Society of Lymphology. *Lymphology.* 2016 Dec;49(4):170-84.

31. Gebruers N, Verbelen H, De Vrieze T, Vos L, Devoogdt N, Fias L, Tjalma W. Current and future perspectives on the evaluation, prevention and conservative management of breast cancer related lymphoedema: A best practice guideline. *Eur J Obstet Gynecol Reprod Biol.* 2017;216:245-253. doi: 10.1016/j.ejogrb.2017.07.035.

32. Thompson B, Gaitatzis K, Janse de Jonge X, Blackwell R, Koelmeyer LA. Manual lymphatic drainage treatment for lymphedema: a systematic review of the literature. *J Cancer Surviv.* 2021 Apr;15(2):244-258. doi: 10.1007/s11764-020-00928-1.

33. Stuiver MM, ten Tusscher MR, Agasi-Idenburg CS, Lucas C, Aaronson NK, Bossuyt PM. Conservative interventions for preventing clinically detectable upper-limb lymphoedema in patients who are at risk of developing lymphoedema after breast cancer therapy. *Cochrane Database Syst Rev.* 2015;13;(2). doi: 10.1002/14651858.CD009765.

34. Ezzo J, Manheimer E, McNeely ML, Howell DM, Weiss R, Johansson KI, Bao T, Bily L, Tuppo CM, Williams AF, Karadibak D. Manual lymphatic drainage for lymphedema following breast cancer treatment. *Cochrane Database Syst Rev.* 2015;21;(5). doi: 10.1002/14651858.CD003475.

35. Huang TW, Tseng SH, Lin CC, Bai CH, Chen CS, Hung CS, et al. Effects of manual lymphatic drainage on breast cancer-related lymphedema: A systematic review and meta-analysis of randomized controlled trials. *World J Surg Oncol.* 2013;11.

36. Tambour M, Holt M, Speyer A, Christensen R, Gram B. Manual lymphatic drainage adds no further volume reduction to Complete Decongestive Therapy on breast cancer-related lymphoedema: a multicentre, randomised, single-blind trial. *Br J Cancer.* 2018;119(10):1215-22.

37. Gradalski T, Ochalek K, Kurpiewska J. Complex Decongestive Lymphatic Therapy with or Without Vodder II Manual Lymph Drainage in More Severe Chronic Postmastectomy Upper Limb Lymphedema: A Randomized Noninferiority Prospective Study. J Pain Symptom Manage. 2015;50(6):750-7.

38. Andersen L, Højris I, Erlandsen M, Andersen J. Treatment of breast-cancer-related lymphedema with or without manual lymphatic drainage--a randomized study. *Acta Oncol.* 2000;39(3):399-405. doi: 10.1080/028418600750013186.

39. *The diagnosis and treatment of peripheral lymphedema: 2020 Consensus Document of the International Society of Lymphology – PubMed. [cited 2020 Sep 16]; Available from: https://pubmed.ncbi.nlm.nih.gov/32521126/*

40. Johansson K, Jönsson C, Björk-Eriksson T. Compression Treatment of Breast Edema: A Randomized Controlled Pilot Study. *Lymphat Res Biol.* 2020;18(2):129-35.

41. Kilbreath SL, Ward LC, Davis GM, Degnim AC, Hackett DA, Skinner TL, Black D. Reduction of breast lymphoedema secondary to breast cancer: a randomised controlled exercise trial. *Breast Cancer Res Treat.* 2020 Nov;184(2):459-467. doi: 10.1007/s10549-020-05863-4.

42. Bloomquist K, Oturai P, Steele ML, Adamsen L, Mkller T, Christensen KB, et al. Heavy-load lifting: Acute response in breast cancer survivors at risk for lymphedema. *Med Sci Sports Exerc.* 2018;50(2):187-95.

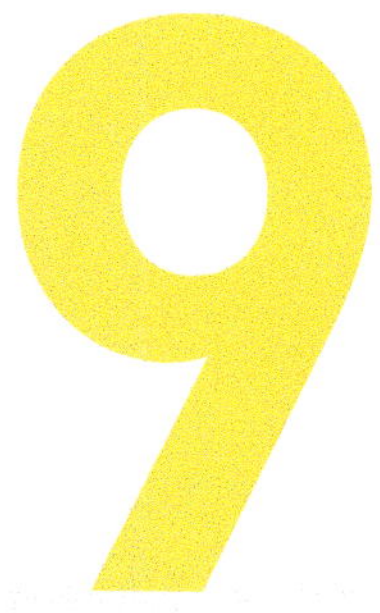 POST-SURGICAL SCARS

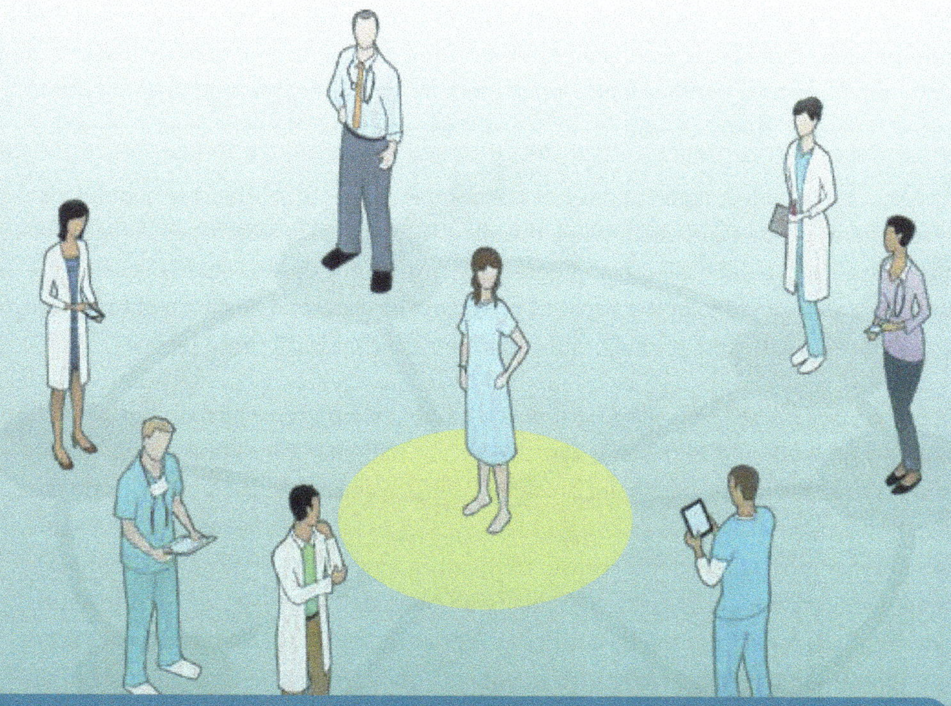

9.1   INTRODUCTION

Surgery can have an enormous impact on a person's life. On top of the emotional reasons (e.g., receiving a diagnosis, having to undergo [urgent] surgery), the aftermath can be very difficult for the patient.

Rehabilitation periods can be long and after that the patient remains with a linear scar, which can be debilitating. The incidence of hypertrophic scarring or problematic scars post-surgery ranges from 40% to 70%.[1] Since the patient is still in the rehabilitation phase at the time of the development of hypertrophic scarring, it is not considered a top priority. However, it has been shown that hypertrophic scars greatly impact the person's quality of life (QoL). More than 50% of patients with skin scars report that it has a negative impact on physical comfort and functioning, acceptability to self and others, social functioning, confidence in the nature and management of their scar and emotional well-being.[2] While follow-up of these hypertrophic scars and their impact on the patient post-surgery is important, it is not systematically done in clinical practice.

The skin is the largest organ of our body. It not only protects us from harm, but it also gives us our unique expression. When the integrity of that skin is damaged, a regenerative process of wound healing commences, which does not always lead to the complete disappearance of scars. In the event of prolonged or disturbed healing a pathological scar is formed with possibly major functional and psychological consequences.

Treatment of scarred skin is a recent development, although we palpate our patients and always work with our hands directly on our patients' skin. Physical therapy for scars is a relatively new treatment modality, and as such knowledge is lacking amongst health practitioners and in scientific research. The overall goal for every health-care practitioner is to help patients recover to their pre-injury state and to strive for an optimal reintegration into society with unaltered potential. To do so, we need to assess and treat our patients in the best possible (evidence-based) way. Assessment of scars is important in the clinical follow-up of patients, for comparative evaluation of treatment modalities and for measuring the efficacy of our interventions. Possible assessment tools will be described as well as interventions. New assessment tools for scars keep emerging. Multiple treatment modalities that were primarily developed for other musculoskeletal or skin disorders have found their way into the treatment of scars, but evidence for their efficacy is frequently lacking.[3]

9.2   FORMATION OF A SCAR

To understand scar formation a good understanding of the anatomy of the skin is essential and is illustrated in figure 9.1. The skin has different layers: the first and most external layer is the epidermis, whose main purpose is to continuously create new cells that move from deep to superficial. The epidermis contains melanocytes that produce melanin via the influence of UV radiation, which causes skin discolouration and pigmentation. The second layer is the dermis, which makes up 90% of the skin and contains hair follicles, blood vessels, sweat glands, etc. The dermis is made up of collagen elastin and extracellular matrix. The deep layer is the hypodermis, which includes the fatty tissue.

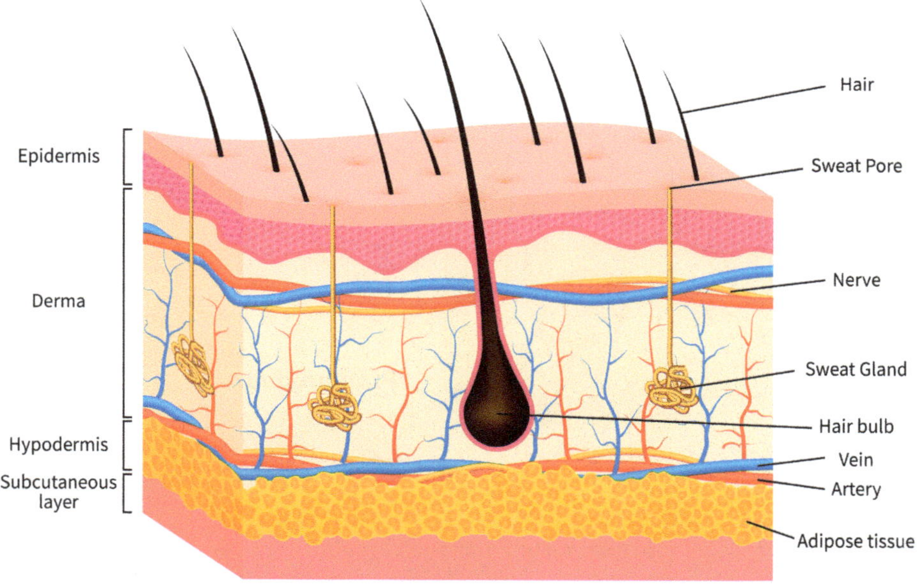

Figure 9.1   Skin anatomy.

Repair of the skin starts within 24-72 hours after injury, with an inflammatory reaction as a first step. The wound is cleaned by white blood cells and vasodilatation in the capillaries causing redness and edema in the skin.[4,5] In a second phase, which may last for up to six weeks (the proliferation or fibroblastic phase), epithelialization, wound contraction and collagen production occur, characterizing the progress in time. Granulation tissue is formed and myofibroblasts (transdifferentiated fibroblasts) play a key role in contraction of the wound edges (closing the wound).[6] The maturation or remodeling phase takes at least one year to complete and is the last step in normal wound healing in which stronger collagen is produced and scar tissue is formed.[4] The different steps in normal wound healing are illustrated in figure 9.2. The presence of myofibroblasts should decrease after wound closure but in hypertrophic scars the myofibroblasts persist[5] with an overabundant deposition of collagen. Various factors like size of the wound, location, infection, age, skin type, health of the patient and mechanical tension may influence normal scar formation and cause hypertrophy.[7] Furthermore, wounds that are not healed within 2-3 weeks and have a prolonged or excessive inflammatory phase[8] are more likely to become hypertrophic scars.[9] Scar maturation may last as long as two years,[10] or even up to 5 years,[11] and besides their aesthetic consequences scars affect functions of the skin like sensation and the capacity to evaporate (due to the diminished sweat glands).

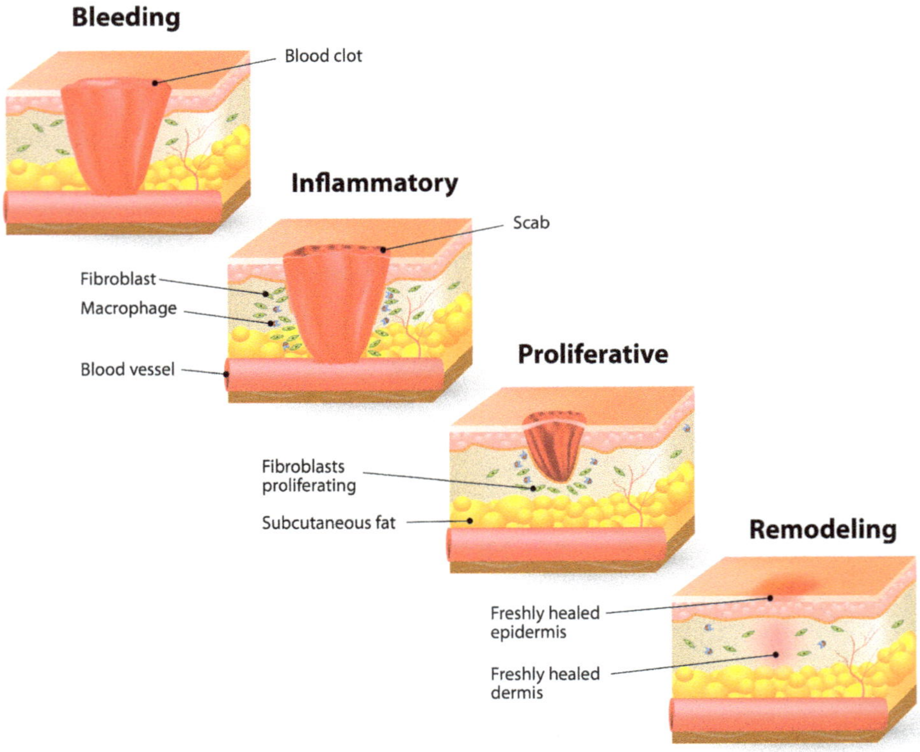

Figure 9.2   Phases of wound healing.

9.3 HYPERTROPHIC SCAR POST-SURGERY/ SCARS AND SCAR CHARACTERISTICS

9.3.1 Scar evolution

In the developed world, it is estimated that each year around 100 million people acquire scars following elective surgery and surgery for trauma.[12] Scars change over time and the resolution of erythema (skin redness) is a key factor in establishing scar maturation. All scars, normal and problematic, evolve from immature to mature scars. Immature scars are visible as erythematous and slightly raised from the surrounding skin surface. Mature scars are flat and colour ranges between white and hyperpigmented. Mature white scars are characterized by the absence of melanocytes and mature hyperpigmented scars are typically manifested in ethnicities with already increased melanocytes in the basal layer of the epidermis.[13]

9.3.2 Scar types

There are many different scar types[14] with different physical features:
- atrophic scars;
- stretched scars;
- hypertrophic scars;
- keloid scars.

9.3.2.1 Atrophic scars

Atrophic scars are typically flat or have indentations compared to the surrounding surface area and lesions are commonly seen as a result of acne.[15]

9.3.2.2 Stretched scars

Stretched scars appear when initially linear surgical scars become widened after surgery, usually occurring in the first three weeks post-surgery.[16]

9.3.2.3 Hypertrophic scars

Hypertrophic scars and keloids are scars with a higher volume that appear raised compared to the surrounding surface and can be distinguished by looking at the boundaries of the original wound. Hypertrophic scars remain within the boundaries of the original wound, whereas keloids tend to expand beyond the original wound boundaries.[17]

A keloid scar appears very voluminous, is mushroom- or cauliflower-shaped and is characterized by the overgrowth that can occur years after the original injury. Keloids occur more in darker skin types (Fitzpatrick skin types 4-6). The pathogenesis and genetics of keloids is complex and involves genetic predisposition.[13] The in-depth assessment and/ or treatment of keloids is beyond the scope of this chapter.

9.3.3   Scar characteristics and appearance

Scar characteristics and appearance are influenced by the cause, depth, size, location, treatment type and genetic predisposition. An abnormal scar can lead to anomalies in skin colour, thickness, pliability or elasticity, texture and contraction.[18] Reducing these scar characteristics is the focus of many scar treatments and most of the first-line treatments have shown merit in reducing thickness, improving colour and making scars more pliable.[19-21]

9.3.4   Scar hypertrophy

Peacock defined a hypertrophic scar as a scar raised above the skin level that stays within the confines of the original lesion.[17] We can make a distinction between hypertrophic linear scars and hypertrophic wide scars.[13] The incidence of hypertrophic scarring varies from 40% to 70%[22] following surgery and from 30% up to 91% following burns.[1,23] Hypertrophic scars may have aesthetic and physical consequences. The red to purple coloured scar, due to increased blood flow in the capillaries, may cause pain, itch, alteration in sensitivity and a decrease in range of motion due to skin reduced pliability (because of the lack of elastin), especially if the scarred skin overlaps a joint.

Wounds subjected to tension due to motion or body location are at increased risk of scar hypertrophy. Specific anatomical locations such as shoulders, neck, sternum, knees and ankles have higher predilection for hypertrophic scar formation.[24] The (re) integration of patients with hypertrophic scars into our society which places an emphasis on external appearance may also cause problems.[25]

The first three months after surgery is the time when remodeling, the last phase of wound healing, is at its peak during a normal wound healing process. While some incisional scars will continue to heal without significant protest and form normotrophic scars, those incisions destined for hypertrophic scar formation will begin to reveal themselves during this period.[26]

To sum up: individual patients may face different scar symptoms and each scar and each patient is different as well as the consequences for the patient. It is imperative to get a good overview of the different symptoms and characteristics over time, which is why a good and in-depth holistic biopsychosocial clinical investigation, along with a thorough anamnesis focused on wound healing and the immature/mature scar, should be part of the post-surgical care process.

9.4 SCARS AND HUMAN FUNCTIONING

Our research has found biopsychosocial dysfunctioning/disability in patients with scars. Refer back to the section on the ICF Framework in Chapter 1 to learn more about functioning/dysfunctioning. Patients who suffer from (post-surgical) hypertrophic scars may thus have aesthetic consequences, but may also be confronted with long-term impairments in **body structures** (e.g., thick/red hypertrophic scar) and **body functioning** (e.g., itch, pain, inelastic scar), **activity limitations** (e.g., lifting objects, inability to write) and **participation restrictions** (e.g., not being able to work/go to school)[3] during their rehabilitation. Dysfunctioning/disability in patients with post-surgical scars will be the main theme of this chapter. An exploration of outcome measures across all levels of the ICF may help to make the very complex consequences more comprehensible.

9.5 OBJECTIVE AND SUBJECTIVE SCAR ASSESSMENTS IN PATIENTS WITH SCARS

Several quantitative and qualitative measurements are needed to quantify scars for the purposes of determining response to treatment and evaluating outcomes. Scar assessments can be objective or subjective. Objective assessments provide a quantitative measurement of the scar, whereas subjective assessments are observer dependent.

The **objective** assessment can evaluate one or more aspects of scar characteristics (impairments in body structures or body functions). Objective scar assessment tools enable comparison of different treatment protocols and allow an objective follow-up and reproducible evaluation of scars. They are essential for scientific studies, for medico-legal purposes and for the clinical follow-up of an individual patient.[27] Below, a few scar parameters will be further explained and elaborated on.

Objective scar assessment tools can provide useful quantitative measurements of physiological or physical scar parameters.

Physiological properties include:

- trans-epidermal water loss (TEWL);
- tactile sensitivity;
- skin hydration.

Physical properties include:

- colour (with erythema and melanin included);
- pliability;
- thickness and topography.[28,29]

Besides erythema, the most important characteristics that provide information about the maturation of hypertrophic scars are TEWL and water content.[27] Scar pliability is one of the most important features in scar assessment.[30] It represents the reduced extensibility of the collagen fibre network and quantifies mechanical tension on scarred skin. The diminished pliability in scarred skin may result in joint immobility and further impact daily living activities and participation. TEWL is an important parameter for evaluating skin barrier function and the efficiency of the skin to retain water. TEWL rates are usually higher in young scars since the skin is disrupted and the stratum corneum barrier functions of the epidermis are damaged. The change in scar thickness, particularly measured with ultrasound tools, has been adopted as one of the objective indicators for assessing the maturation of hypertrophic scars. Ultrasound imaging is a non-invasive, reliable and convenient method for visualizing epidermal and dermal thickness and density. To sum up, there are a variety of objective measures for assessing scar characteristics over time and many reviews and studies are available. Choosing an objective scar assessment tool is usually based on the scar characteristic central to the research being performed.[31] Assessment of objective scar parameters has proven to be valuable in developing new treatment strategies, but less in the clinical context, and more importantly it does not take into account the patient's perception of the scar.[31] Therefore, an adequate patient-oriented assessment of physical scar features is crucial as part of the clinical evaluation and follow-up of scars, in defining scar treatment options for the patient and for medico-legal reasons (e.g., for reimbursement of treatment and proof of disability).[32,33] To fill this gap, subjective scar assessment by the use of questionnaires or scales has been developed by several researchers.

As already stated, several reviews are available[18,24,34-36] on non-invasive objective and subjective assessments of hypertrophic scars, but few instruments have investigated physical features of scars across a variety of scar types.[34] The majority of the available literature on TEWL, colour and other scar measurement tools were tested on post-burn scars.[34] How transferable these data would be on other scar types remains uncertain.

Besides objective scar assessments, subjective scar scales and Patient Reported Outcome Measures are important and show the impact of the scar and the different treatments on areas of health and functioning that are important to the person with scars.

9.6 PATIENT-REPORTED OUTCOME MEASURES FOR SCARS IN CLINICAL PRACTICE

9.6.1 Scar scales

In patient-centred care and taking into account that we need to measure what is important for our patients, PROMs can be used to get an idea of their dysfunction. Scar scales focus on scar characteristics and can be patient-reported or clinician-reported. The first scar scale was described in 1978 and included an assessment of colour, thickness and density. Since then, more than thirty scar scales have been developed, but the best known and most used are certainly the Vancouver Scar Scale (VSS), with all its modifications, and the Patient and Observer Scar Assessment Scale (POSAS).[30] The VSS is pioneer work and is in fact not a scale and can only be used for burn scars.

The POSAS questionnaire was created in 2004. This is a short and yet comprehensive scale, applicable to all types of scars. It is a scar scale that measures scar quality and contains a section that patients can score. It consists of six items (one for each characteristic) and an additional score for the general impression and some categories. Taking a broader view, the POSAS is suitable for both single-moment and longitudinal evaluation. In terms of content, the POSAS has the PROM (itching and pain). Literature describes the use of the POSAS in children from 12 years of age and in adults. It is applicable to both men and women. In terms of use post burn, it seems to be used for scars between three months and thirty years old. One of the biggest advantages is that the POSAS only takes 5 minutes to administer.

A recent review on PROMs for surgical and traumatic scars stated that there is only one patient-reported scar scale[33] that measures scar quality, the POSAS. The Manchester Scar Scale (MSS), the Stony Brook Scar Evaluation Scale (SBSES), the Patient-Reported Impact of Scars Measure (PRISM) and the Patient Scar Assessment Questionnaire (PSAQ) are several other scar scales or questionnaires that include items on QoL or satisfaction,[30] in addition to items on scar quality.

The POSAS assesses physical scar features and scar appearance[37] and has the added benefit of capturing patient ratings in comparison to the VSS and was proven more reliable than the latter.[30,31] The POSAS includes subjective ratings for pain, itch, colour, stiffness, thickness and relief (all impairments in BS or BF), using the Patient Scar Assessment Scale (PSAS). The observer rates vascularity, pigmentation, thickness, relief, pliability and surface area with the Observer Scar Assessment Scale (OSAS). The POSAS is a reliable and valid scale for measuring scar quality[33,37] and is applicable to various scar types.[33] It is a very short and feasible scar scale and is downloadable together with its user instructions from the POSAS website (www.POSAS.org). An updated version of the POSAS is expected soon.

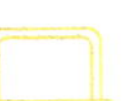 You can find a link to the downloadable POSAS scar scale and its user instructions on the online learning platform Sofia.

9.6.2   QoL measures

The main goal of QoL measures is to describe the burden of disease of the population studied. QoL instruments focus on activities and participation, which are considered to be the components most relevant to patients and society, and are applicable to all health conditions. These instruments make it possible to compare functioning and health across health conditions, populations and interventions.[38]

It has been demonstrated that the QoL of patients with skin conditions (including patients with pathologic scarring) is as much reduced as that of patients with severe heart failure or diabetes mellitus.[39,40] Accordingly, it is crucial that the well-being and QoL of patients with skin conditions be evaluated.

Expert consensus exists on using both generic and disease-specific QoL questionnaires to capture the full impact of a health condition and because the specific measures are often more responsive to change in that specific population.[41] In patients with scars following injury or surgery, QoL can be assessed with the Dermatology Life Quality Index (DLQI)[42], a specific tool that has shown promising results and significant differences in the impact on QoL between different scar type groups.[43] The DLQI[42] is the most commonly used dermatology-specific QoL measure in clinical trials.[44] Within the scar population it is also one of the most commonly used QoL questionnaires. The brevity and simplicity of the DLQI is an explanation for the popularity of the measures, both clinically and within research. Within the scar population the generic European Quality of Life-5 Dimensions (EQ-5D) is one of the most frequently used QoL measures.[45] It includes relevant health domains, is applicable in all kinds of injury populations and in widely different age ranges, provides a link to utility scores and has several practical advantages (e.g., brevity, availability in different languages).[3] When selecting QoL measures for clinical studies or for clinical practice one can consider the ICF-based comparison of the QoL measures in order to establish what should be measured. The generic measures can capture comorbidities, allow comparison across conditions and are useful for cost-effectiveness analyses.

To capture the full spectrum of functioning of a person with hypertrophic scars, a combination of questionnaires and subjective or objective scar assessments seems obligatory.[3,46] From our experience the combination of the POSAS, DLQI and a generic QoL measure (e.g. EQ-5D) are easily administered and widely accessible questionnaires with good psychometric properties to allow patient-centred evaluation of the scar impact.

The PSAS, the Bock Quality of Life Questionnaire for Patients with Keloids and Hypertrophic Scars (Bock), the PRISM and the PSAQ are four PROMs that have been developed specifically for surgical and traumatic scars. The PRISM assesses QoL and physical symptoms, but both the PRISM and the Bock lack appearance domains.[32]

We recommend repeating holistic assessments/evaluations at regular time intervals. A recent article identified key subthemes that contribute to the overarching theme of patient-centred scar assessment:
- patient-led care;
- continuity in care;
- learning how to self-manage scarring;
- psychological assessment.

The article also highlighted the necessity to state and explain the purpose of objective scar measures and/or subjective scar scales that are being used. In the care process, reviewing with the patients the completed scales and results of objective testing may aid in the holistic view of scar progression and assist unexperienced patients in understanding their scar symptomology.[47]

Validity, reliability and responsiveness are important measurement properties which must be evaluated prior to using an objective scar measure: a scale for scar assessments or a QoL measure.

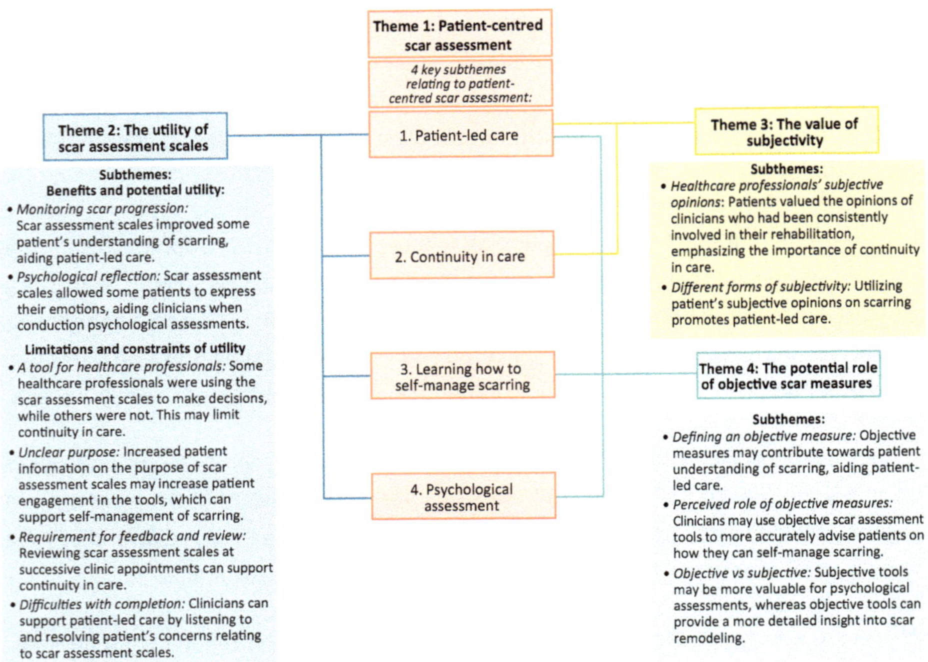

Source: Kate Price et al.[47]

Figure 9.3 Diagram illustrating links between the four key subthemes of patient-centred scar assessment and other themes which describe scar assessment strategies.

For clinical evaluations of the patient with post-surgical scars in a clinical setting, figure 9.4 shows an ICF form with aspects and outcome measures to consider. This form cannot be considered as complete since it may lack other relevant items. It was formulated to visualize the aspects discussed above and created from experience with investigated measures. It encompasses different aspects within ICF domains that may be clinically feasible to assess.

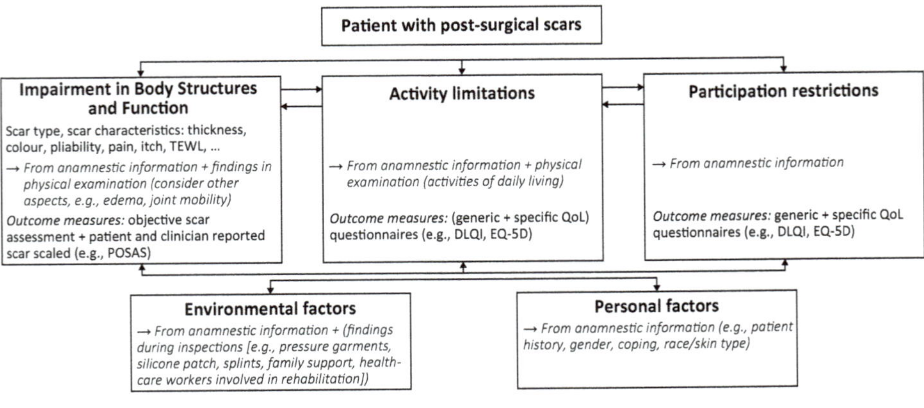

Figure 9.4 ICF form with an overview of relevant aspects of ICF domains to assess in patients with post-surgical scars, together with associated outcome measures.

9.7 SCAR TREATMENTS

A wide variety of non-invasive (e.g., compression, silicone, massage), semi-invasive (e.g., laser, micro-needling) and invasive scar treatments (surgical excision) exist and advancements in semi-invasive treatments such as laser treatment and micro-needling seem promising.

Our scar treatments as physiotherapists consist mainly of non-invasive skin techniques: with our hands we move, manipulate and/or fold the skin with the aim of making it more supple and preventing it from done in combination with other therapies (e.g., pressure therapy, silicone). Combination therapies are needed to achieve a good scar outcome. These scar treatments must be considered in addition to the typical post-surgical rehabilitation aimed at strength/mobility/improving the activities of the daily living, etc. Depending on the size, scar age, body location, origin of the scar and the wish of the patient, we have to adjust our scar treatment and choose the best treatment which almost always consists of a combination of different treatments.

9.8 GUIDELINES AND PREVENTIVE MEASURES FOR POST-SURGICAL SCARS

To date, it remains much more efficient to prevent excessive scars than to treat them. The most successful treatment of a hypertrophic scar or keloid is achieved when the scar is immature but the overlying epithelium is intact.[48] The classical non-invasive treatment and preventive options are numerous. An international, multidisciplinary group of 24 experts developed a set of practical guidelines based only on expert opinion for the management of linear, hypertrophic and keloid scars. These were created for surgeons, dermatologists, general practitioners and other physicians and health-care workers involved in the prevention and the treatment of scars.[49]

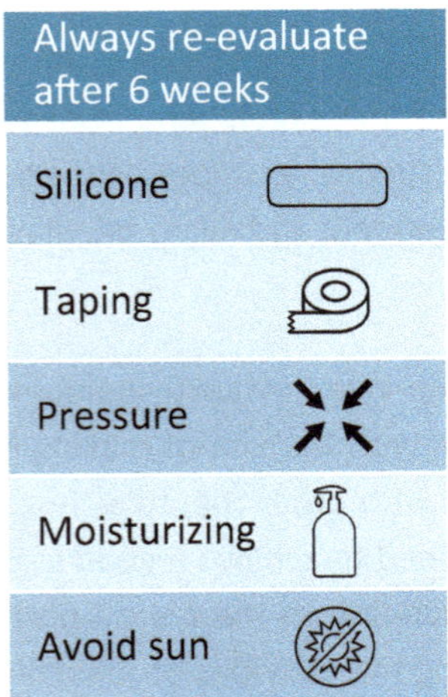

Source: adapted from Monstrey et al.[49]

Figure 9.5   Practical guidelines for optimal linear post-surgical scars.

Following surgery the first priority should always be the prevention of abnormal scar formation. Excessive scar formation can also be prevented by a wide range of measures that reduce inflammation and provide rapid wound closure, reducing the risk of infection through rinsing and disinfection and optimal dressings providing moist wound healing and/or early surgical wound coverage. These measures are already common practice in post-surgical wound management. The major components of scar prevention immediately after wound closure are as follows:

- tension relief;
- hydration;
- tension-reducing taping;
- occlusion;
- pressure garments, if possible.

Wounds that have greater tension have a higher risk of developing excessive scarring.[16] This can be reduced by the use of post-surgical paper taping for a three-month period. A stress-shielding device can reduce mechanical stress, reduce tension and prevent and reduce excessive scar formation.[50] Moisturizing emollient, creams and dressings retaining moisture such as silicone gel sheets and fluid silicone gel can reduce the size and pain or discomfort associated with scars and improve their appearance. Moreover, they diminish itching in scars. After wound healing, water still evaporates more rapidly through scar tissue compared to healthy skin and this may take over a year to recover.[51] Silicone products help to prevent excessive scar formation by restoring the water barrier by means of their occlusive nature together with hydration of the stratum corneum of the epidermis. Silicones need to be used as soon as the suture is healed.[52] The use of topical silicone for the prevention and treatment of hypertrophic scarring was first introduced in 1981 by Perkins et al. to treat scars. Silicone has since been used in various forms, including silicone gel, silicone gel sheets[53] and silicone sprays. Various randomized clinical studies, also in relation to our work, have demonstrated that silicone gel has a positive effect on the healing process of hypertrophic scars.[54,55]

Pressure garments are indicated for more widespread scarring, especially for burn scars,[49] but are not used in clinical practice to prevent post-surgical hypertrophic scars. This is probably because thescar is relatively small compared to a large pressure garment (e.g., pants, jacket), which is very unpractical, expensive and uncomfortable for the patient. Since pressure garments are not always easy to apply and are primarily indicated for existing hypertrophy and more widespread scarring this strategy is beyond the scope of this chapter.

Expert consensus exists on the ideal and best supported evidence for scar prevention in the first three months but no RCTs are available for post-surgical scar prevention. Optimal prevention for linear scars involves avoiding sun exposure, hydration, the use of silicone and taping. This is displayed in figure 9.5.[49] Silicone is the gold standard non-invasive, first-line prophylactic treatment option with the best supported evidence.

9.9 NON-INVASIVE PHYSICAL TREATMENTS FOR HYPERTROPHIC SCARS

Physical scar management – including manual and mechanical skin techniques – are currently being used clinically in physiotherapeutic treatments, although evidence-based guidelines (based on good quality randomized clinical trials [RCT]) on physiotherapeutic skin treatments are lacking for the prevention and treatment of scars.

Pain and pruritus significantly improve with massage therapy and also objective measures on thickness, melanin, erythema, TEWL and elasticity showed promising results from massage therapy.[57] Massage therapy seems to have positive effects on patient's perspectives and scar characteristics, although the proof for this is limited. The few studies that have been written had small sample sizes, sometimes only used subjective measures and no clear explanation of the exact massage therapy, timing and or frequency was described.

In the first months after wound closure, given the fragility of the skin, physical scar treatments must take into account the changed characteristics of this 'young' immature scarred skin. But also in the longer run, the choice of therapy modalities and parameters must be done with caution, as a scar can remain active for up to two years after its formation with remodeling.

Moisturizing lotions, whether applied with or without massage, are essential in scar aftercare with the aim of restoring the skin barrier. This form of hydration is therefore recommended to all patients, even several times a day. Furthermore, in clinical practice on immature scars, we also use very gentle skin massage techniques like skin gliding (glissements) or skin folding involving lifting the skinand a skin fold technique (alongement) to counteract adhesion to the lower layer and hypertrophy. For younger immature scars, movements of low intensity and frequency are recommended, whereas older mature scars can be treated with more intensive soft tissue mobilization techniques like the splitting up technique: creating a skin fold by lifting the skin and slowly mobilizing this skin fold in a slow and gentle manner (fractionnement). It is important to avoid friction on the skin. Traditionally, scar massage is done with a cream medium, but for the above mentioned manual scar techniques no creams are advised to allow a good palpation and grasp on the scarred skin.

Massage on scarred skin reduces pain and itching, and shows improvement in skin thickness, redness, water permeability and elasticity. Massage is practiced worldwide, yet the evidence for its improvement of scars is weak. The limited studies that have investigated the effects are of poor quality. Different massage various massage applications are described and the effects could possibly be explained by the creams or lotions that were used during massage treatments.

Vacuum massage (or depressomassage or endermology) is a non-invasive mechanical massage technique. The treatment head of the machine creates a skin fold (with negative pressure or suction) that can be manipulated. Although the vacuum massage was invented to treat traumatic burn scars, few studies on its effects on burn scars or post-surgical scars can be found. A review on the physiological effects of vacuum massage found evidence of collagen restructuring and remodelling[58]; however, the studies included in the review were of poor methodologic quality, not performed in humans or not performed on (burn) scars. It remains to be proven whether the described physiological efficacy of vacuum massage can be seen in burn and/or post-surgical linear scars. A comparative study found limited evidence of the improvement of colour and TEWL for vacuum massage therapy as an addition to standard of care (hydration, pressure garment, silicone and physical therapy). This modality might be considered as an additional non-invasive treatment. Very few studies investigated the effects of vacuum massage on human models with scars. The heterogeneous population and the wide diversity of study designs make it very hard to translate the results to the post-surgical scars population in humans.

Extracorporal shockwave therapy (ESWT) has shown its value in wound healing and as an additional treatment modality in the first three months after wound closure. A randomized controlled trial showed improved elasticity for young hypertrophic burn scars with just one treatment per week and 10 treatments in total.[56] This non-invasive scar treatment is safe, well tolerated by patients, has low associated complication rates, is easy to apply, cost-effective and can be used in an outpatient setting.

9.10 MECHANOTHERAPY

In recent years there has been an increasing interest in the mechanobiology of scars. The influence of mechanical forces on skin has been examined since 1861, when Langer first reported the existence of lines of tension in cadaver skin.[59] Internal tension in the dermis leads to cell – extracellular matrix and cell – cell interactions that transfers external mechanical forces into biochemical signals inside the cell.[60] Khan et al. introduced the term 'mechanotherapy' and presented the current scientific knowledge underpinning how mechanical load may be used therapeutically to stimulate tissue repair and remodelling.[61] Recent developments in mechanobiology have illuminated the effects of physical forces on cells and tissues and have led to the realization that 'the old physical therapy model' should be updated. Recent studies showed how mechanotherapy target particular cells, molecules and tissues. The role of mechanical force in various therapies, including microdeformating soft tissue techniques, shockwave, vacuum massage, tissue expansion, skin stretching and tension-reducing therapies, is the subject of numerous ongoing clinical trials.[62,63] It can be assumed that many of the physical scar management methods, including compression therapy, manual skin techniques/scar massage, silicone therapy, adhesive tension reducing tape and occlusive dressing therapy, are related to mechanotransduction mechanisms.

Mechanical forces is the subject of growing interest amongst medical researchers. Mechanotherapy or the employment of mechanical means for the cure of disease has had several definitions and involves physical therapy (e.g., massage therapy and orthopedic rehabilitation).[63] It has been suggested that physical therapy helps in healing or the homeostasis of tissue outside the musculoskeletal system and may be able to oppose specific pathophysiology and diseases. Recently, mechanotherapy has been redefined as a therapeutic intervention that reduces and reverses injury to damaged tissue or promotes the homeostasis of healthy tissue by mechanical means at the molecular, cellular or tissue level.[63]

All skin/scar techniques (manual and mechanical) techniques like manual defibrosing massage techniques, shockwave therapy and vacuum massage work according to that same principle of mechanotherapy,with the aim of restructuring the collagen network in the scar tissue and reducing the impairments in body structures (thick, red scar) and impairments in functioning (e.g., inelastic, itchy, painful scar).

Pressure garments and silicone therapy are the most widely known evidence-based conservative treatments for hypertrophic scars after a burn injury.[52,64] These treatment modalities are recommended in the European Burn Association Practice Guidelines, are part of recent scar management recommendations[65] and are considered as standard of care in the physical treatments of hypertrophic scars at Oscare, an after-care and research centre for patients with (burn) scars. Both pressure and silicone therapy are subsequently included in the usual care treatment. The in-depth investigation of these treatments is beyond the scope of this chapter.

As already stated, the effect of non-invasive treatment for (non-burn) hypertrophic scars remains understudied. Several techniques for scars were proven to be effective through extensive use[66] but no optimal treatment method has been established.[36] Vacuum massage may prove its use beyond the burn population but needs to be further investigated.

The review and updated 'Scar Management Practical Guidelines: Non-invasive and invasive measures' by Monstrey at al. includes ideal preventive strategies for linear scars and more widespread scars.[49] Knowledge of these preventive strategies and their implementation within clinical practice is necessary in the effort to avoid abnormal scar formation and strive for a scarless world.

For clinical practice and research purposes, the assessment of scars with objective and subjective measures and scales or questionnaires allows us to assess changes over time, demonstrate the effects of therapies and compare scars with each other. They are indispensable for evaluating scarred patients and for demonstrating the effects of new forms of therapy. With the patient at the centre of scar aftercare, it is important that the patient's perception is included. A holistic approach to the patient with a good interview and establishing the patient's request for help or patient preferences is essential for steering the therapeutic process. The various therapies described here are still under further development and investigation. From the experiences and findings to date, we can conclude that the therapies (massage, shockwave and taping) for immature scars should be applied in a dosed and slow manner. The treatments should be carried out with a good understanding of the underlying mechanisms and effects. Which therapy is most suitable for which type of scar, as well as which duration, frequency and intensity of the various therapies are ideal, are challenges for the future. For each scar characteristics, specific (combinations of) non-invasive treatment options are possible.

On the online learning platform Sofia, you can find a link to a website that aims to give an overview of all treatment options for improving scars.

9.11 REFERENCES

1. Lewis WHP, Sun KKY. Hypertrophic scar: a genetic hypothesis. Burns. 1990;16(3):176-178. doi:10.1016/0305-4179(90)90033-S
2. Brown BC, McKenna SP, Siddhi K, McGrouther DA, Bayat A. The hidden cost of skin scars: quality of life after skin scarring. J Plast Reconstr Aesthetic Surg. 2008;61(9):1049-1058. doi:10.1016/j.bjps.2008.03.020
3. Meirte J. The ICF as a Framework for Post Burn Dysfunctioning: Evaluation, Quality of Life and Vacuum Massage in Patients with Hypertrophic Burn Scars.; 2016.
4. Hardy MA. The biology of scar formation. Phys Ther. 1989;69(12):1014-1024. doi:10.1093/ptj/69.12.1014
5. Junker JPE, Kratz C, Tollbäck A, Kratz G. Mechanical tension stimulates the transdifferentiation of fibroblasts into myofibroblasts in human burn scars. Burns. 2008;34(7):942-946. doi:10.1016/j.burns.2008.01.010
6. Desmoulière A, Chaponnier C, Gabbiani G. Tissue repair, contraction, and the myofibroblast. Wound Repair Regen. 13(1):7-12. doi:10.1111/j.1067-1927.2005.130102.x
7. Mustoe TA. Scars and keloids. BMJ. 2004;328(7452):1329-1330. doi:10.1136/bmj.328.7452.1329
8. Wong VW, Paterno J, Sorkin M, et al. Mechanical force prolongs acute inflammation via T-cell-dependent pathways during scar formation. FASEB J. 2011;25(12):4498-4510. doi:10.1096/fj.10-178087
9. Monstrey S, Hoeksema H, Verbelen J, Pirayesh A, Blondeel P. Assessment of burn depth and burn wound healing potential. Burns. 2008;34(6):761-769. doi:10.1016/j.burns.2008.01.009
10. Hellström M, Hellström S, Engström-Laurent A, Bertheim U. The structure of the basement membrane zone differs between keloids, hypertrophic scars and normal skin: a possible background to an impaired function. J Plast Reconstr Aesthet Surg. 2014;67(11):1564-1572. doi:10.1016/j.bjps.2014.06.014

11. Kant S, Van Den Kerckhove E, Colla C, Van Der Hulst R, De Grzymala AP. Duration of Scar Maturation: Retrospective Analyses of 361 Hypertrophic Scars over 5 Years. Adv Ski Wound Care. 2019;32(1):26-34. doi:10.1097/01.ASW.0000547415.38888.c4

12. Sund B. New Developments in Wound Care. London: PJB Publications; 2000.

13. Mustoe TA. International Scar Classification in 2019. In: Textbook on Scar Management.; 2020:79-84. doi:10.1007/978-3-030-44766-3

14. Bayat A, McGrouther DA, Ferguson MWJ. Skin scarring. BMJ. 2003;326(7380):88-92.

15. Tsao SS, Dover JS, Arndt KA, Kaminer MS. Scar management: keloid, hypertrophic, atrophic, and acne scars. Semin Cutan Med Surg. 2002;21(1):46-75. doi:10.1016/s1085-5629(02)80719-2

16. Sommerlad BC, Creasey JM. The stretched scar: a clinical and histological study. Br J Plast Surg. 1978;31(1):34-45. doi:10.1016/0007-1226(78)90012-7

17. Peacock EE, Madden JW, Trier WC. Biologic basis for the treatment of keloids and hypertrophic scars. South Med J. 1970;63(7):755-760.

18. van Zuijlen PPM, Angeles AP, Kreis RW, Bos KE, Middelkoop E. Scar assessment tools: implications for current research. Plast Reconstr Surg. 2002;109(3):1108-1122. doi:10.1097/00006534-200203000-00052

19. Ahn ST, Monafo WW, Mustoe TA. Topical silicone gel: a new treatment for hypertrophic scars. Surgery. 1989;106(4):781-786; discussion 786-7. http://www.ncbi.nlm.nih.gov/pubmed/2529659.

20. Ahn ST, Monafo WW, Mustoe TA. Topical silicone gel for the prevention and treatment of hypertrophic scar. Arch Surg. 1991;126(4):499-504. doi:10.1001/archsurg.1991.01410280103016

21. Li-Tsang CWP, Lau JCM, Choi J, Chan CCC, Jianan L. A prospective randomized clinical trial to investigate the effect of silicone gel sheeting (Cica-Care) on post-traumatic hypertrophic scar among the Chinese population. Burns. 2006;32(6):678-683. doi:10.1016/j.burns.2006.01.016

22. Deitch EA, Wheelahan TM, Rose MP, Clothier J, Cotter J. Hypertrophic burn scars: analysis of variables. J Trauma. 1983;23(10):895-898.

23. Li-Tsang CWP, Lau JCM, Chan CCH. Prevalence of hypertrophic scar formation and its characteristics among the Chinese population. Burns. 2005;31(5):610-616. doi:10.1016/j.burns.2005.01.022

24. Gauglitz G, Korting H, Pavicic T. Hypertrophic scarring and keloids: pathomechanisms and current and emerging treatment strategies. Mol. ... 2011;25(12):629. doi:10.2119/molmed.2009.00153

25. Van Loey NEE, Van Son MJM. Psychopathology and psychological problems in patients with burn scars: epidemiology and management. Am J Clin Dermatol. 2003;4(4):245-272. doi:10.2165/00128071-200304040-00004

26. Son D, Harijan A. Overview of surgical scar prevention and management. J Korean Med Sci. 2014;29(6):751-757. doi:10.3346/jkms.2014.29.6.751

27. Brusselaers N, Pirayesh A, Hoeksema H, Verbelen J, Blot S, Monstrey S. Burn scar assessment: A systematic review of objective scar assessment tools. Burns. 2010;36(8):1157-1164. doi:10.1016/j.burns.2010.03.016

28. Fell M, Meirte J, Anthonissen M, Maertens K, Pleat J, Moortgat P. The Scarbase Duo®: Intra-rater and inter-rater reliability and validity of a compact dual scar assessment tool. Burns. 2016;42(2):336-344. doi:10.1016/j.burns.2015.08.005

29. Jaspers MEH, Moortgat P. Objective Assessment Techniques: Physiological Parameters in Scar Assessment. In: Textbook on Scar Management.; 2020:149-158. doi:10.1007/978-3-030-44766-3

30. Carrière ME, Kwa KAA, de Haas LEM, et al. Systematic Review on the Content of Outcome Measurement Instruments on Scar Quality. Plast Reconstr surgery Glob open. 2019;7(9):e2424. doi:10.1097/GOX.0000000000002424

31. Tyack Z, Simons M, Spinks A, Wasiak J. A systematic review of the quality of burn scar rating scales for clinical and research use. Burns. 2012;38(1):6-18. doi:10.1016/j.burns.2011.09.021

32. Tyack Z, Wasiak J, Spinks A, Kimble R, Simons M. A guide to choosing a burn scar rating scale for clinical or research use. Burns. 2013;9.

33. Mundy LR, Miller HC, Klassen AF, Cano SJ, Pusic AL. Patient-Reported Outcome Instruments for Surgical and Traumatic Scars: A Systematic Review of their Development, Content, and Psychometric Validation. Aesthetic Plast Surg. 2016;40(5):792-800. doi:10.1007/s00266-016-0642-9

34. Perry DM, McGrouther DA, Bayat A. Current Tools for Noninvasive Objective Assessment of Skin Scars. Plast Reconstr Surg. 2010;126(3):912-923. doi:10.1097/PRS.0b013e3181e6046b

35. Fearmonti R, Bond J, Erdmann D, Levinson H. A review of scar scales and scar measuring devices. Eplasty. 2010;10:e43. http://www.ncbi.nlm.nih.gov/pubmed/20596233.

36. Atiyeh BS. Nonsurgical Management of Hypertrophic Scars: Evidence-Based Therapies, Standard Practices, and Emerging Methods. Aesthetic Plast Surg. 2007;31(5):468-492. doi:10.1007/s00266-006-0253-y

37. Draaijers LJ, Tempelman FRH, Botman Y a. M, et al. The patient and observer scar assessment scale: a reliable and feasible tool for scar evaluation. Plast Reconstr Surg. 2004;113(7):1960-1965; discussion 1966-7. doi:10.1097/01.PRS.0000122207.28773.56

38. Stucki A, Borchers M, Stucki G, Cieza A, Amann E, Ruof J. Content comparison of health status measures for obesity based on the international classification of functioning, disability and health. Int J Obes (Lond). 2006;30(12):1791-1799. doi:10.1038/sj.ijo.0803335

39. Rapp SR, Feldman SR, Exum ML, Fleischer AB, Reboussin DM. Patients with psoriasis reported reduction in physical functioning and mental functioning comparable to that seen in cancer, arthritis, hypertension, heart disease, diabetes, and depression. J Am Acad Dermatol. 1999;41(3 Pt 1):401-407.

40. Bock O, Schmid-Ott G, Malewski P, Mrowietz U. Quality of life of patients with keloid and hypertrophic scarring. Arch Dermatol Res. 2006;297(10):433-438. doi:10.1007/s00403-006-0651-7

41. Wiebe S, Guyatt G, Weaver B, Matijevic S, Sidwell C. Comparative responsiveness of generic and specific quality-of-life instruments. J Clin Epidemiol. 2003;56(1):52-60. doi:10.1016/S0895-4356(02)00537-1

42. Finlay AY, Khan GK. Dermatology Life Quality Index (DLQI)--a simple practical measure for routine clinical use. Clin Exp Dermatol. 1994;19(3):210-216.

43. Reinholz M, Poetschke J, Schwaiger H, Epple A, Ruzicka T, Gauglitz GG. The dermatology life quality index as a means to assess life quality in patients with different scar types. J Eur Acad Dermatology Venereol. 2015;29(11):2112-2119. doi:10.1111/jdv.13135

44. Basra MKA, Fenech R, Gatt RM, Salek MS, Finlay AY. The Dermatology Life Quality Index 1994-2007: a comprehensive review of validation data and clinical results. Br J Dermatol. 2008;159(5):997-1035. doi:10.1111/j.1365-2133.2008.08832.x

45. Meirte J, Van Loey NEE, Maertens K, Moortgat P, Hubens G, Van Daele U. Classification of quality of life subscales within the ICF framework in burn research: Identifying overlaps and gaps. Burns. 2014;40(7). doi:10.1016/j.burns.2014.01.015

46. Meirte J, Van Daele U, Maertens K, Moortgat P, Deleus R, Van Loey NE. Convergent and discriminant validity of quality of life measures used in burn populations. Burns. 2017;43(1):84-92. doi:10.1016/j.burns.2016.07.001

47. Price K, Moiemen N, Nice L, Mathers J. Patient experience of scar assessment and the use of scar assessment tools during burns rehabilitation: a qualitative study. Burn Trauma. 2021;9:1-13. doi:10.1093/burnst/tkab005

48. Mustoe TA, Cooter RD, Gold MH, et al. International clinical recommendations on scar management. Plast Reconstr Surg. 2002;110(2):560-571. doi:10.1097/00006534-200208000-00031

49. Monstrey S, Middelkoop E, Vranckx JJ, et al. Updated scar management practical guidelines: non-invasive and invasive measures. J Plast Reconstr Aesthet Surg. 2014;67(8):1017-1025. doi:10.1016/j.bjps.2014.04.011

50. Gurtner GC, Dauskardt RH, Wong VW, et al. Improving cutaneous scar formation by controlling the mechanical environment: large animal and phase I studies. Ann Surg. 2011;254(2):217-225. doi:10.1097/SLA.0b013e318220b159

51. Suetake T, Sasai S, Zhen YX, Ohi T, Tagami H. Functional analyses of the stratum corneum in scars. Sequential studies after injury and comparison among keloids, hypertrophic scars, and atrophic scars. Arch Dermatol. 1996;132(12):1453-1458. http://www.ncbi.nlm.nih.gov/pubmed/8961874.

52. Mustoe TA. Evolution of silicone therapy and mechanism of action in scar management. Aesthetic Plast Surg. 2008;32(1):82-92. doi:10.1007/s00266-007-9030-9

53. Perkins K, Davey RB, Wallis KA. Silicone gel: a new treatment for burn scars and contractures. Burns Incl Therm Inj. 1983;9(3):201-204. doi:10.1016/0305-4179(83)90039-6

54. Moortgat P, Meirte J, Maertens K, Lafaire C, De Cuyper L, Anthonissen M. Can a Cohesive Silicone Bandage Outperform an Adhesive Silicone Gel Sheet in the Treatment of Scars? A Randomized Comparative Trial. Plast Reconstr Surg. 2019;143(3):902-911. doi:10.1097/PRS.0000000000005369

55. Majàn JIC. Evaluation of a self-adherent soft silicone dressing for the treatment of hypertrophic postoperative scars. J Wound Care. 2006;15(5):193-196. doi:10.12968/jowc.2006.15.5.26913

56. Moortgat P, Anthonissen M, Van Daele U, et al. The effects of shock wave therapy applied on hypertrophic burn scars: a randomised controlled trial. Scars, Burn Heal. 2020;6:205951312097562. doi:10.1177/2059513120975624

57. Cho YS, Jeon JH, Hong A, et al. The effect of burn rehabilitation massage therapy on hypertrophic scar after burn: a randomized controlled trial. Burns. 2014;40(8):1513-1520. doi:10.1016/j.burns.2014.02.005

58. Meirte J, Moortgat P, Anthonissen M, et al. Short-term effects of vacuum massage on epidermal and dermal thickness and density in burn scars: an experimental study. Burn Trauma. 2016;4(1):27. doi:10.1186/s41038-016-0052-x

59. Silver FH, Siperko LM, Seehra GP. Mechanobiology of force transduction in dermal tissue. Skin Res Technol. 2003;9(1):3-23. doi:10.1034/j.1600-0846.2003.00358.x

60. Ingber DE. Cellular mechanotransduction: putting all the pieces together again. FASEB J. 2006;20(7):811-827. doi:10.1096/fj.05-5424rev

61. Khan KM, Scott A. Mechanotherapy: how physical therapists' prescription of exercise promotes tissue repair. Br J Sports Med. 2009;43(4):247-252. doi:10.1136/bjsm.2008.054239

62. Frairia R, Berta L. Biological effects of extracorporeal shock waves on fibroblasts. A review. Muscles Ligaments Tendons J. 2011;1(4):138-147. http://www.ncbi.nlm.nih.gov/pubmed/23738262.

63. Huang C, Holfeld J, Schaden W, Orgill D, Ogawa R. Mechanotherapy: revisiting physical therapy and recruiting mechanobiology for a new era in medicine. Trends Mol Med. 2013;19(9):555-564. doi:10.1016/j.molmed.2013.05.005

64. Anzarut A, Olson J, Singh P, Rowe BH, Tredget EE. The effectiveness of pressure garment therapy for the prevention of abnormal scarring after burn injury: a meta-analysis. J Plast Reconstr Aesthetic Surg. 2009;62(1):77-84. doi:10.1016/j.bjps.2007.10.052

65. Gold MH, McGuire M, Mustoe TA, et al. Updated international clinical recommendations on scar management: Part 2 – Algorithms for scar prevention and treatment. Dermatologic Surg. 2014;40(8):825-831. doi:10.1111/dsu.0000000000000050

66. Heppt M, Breuninger H, Reinholz M, Feller-Heppt G, Ruzicka T, Gauglitz G. Current Strategies in the Treatment of Scars and Keloids. Facial Plast Surg. 2015;31(04):386-395. doi:10.1055/s-0035-1563694